The

Young Adult Chronic Patient

Collected Articles From H&CP

CONTENTS

COMMENTARY

THE EMERGING CRISIS IN CHRONIC CARE

It is ironic that, following a period of intense interest in the plight of the chronically mentally ill who have been dumped from large state institutions into largely nonexistent "communities," we now face a new crisis—a tremendous increase in their numbers due to population changes. Morton Kramer, D.Sc., longtime head of the Division of Biometrics and Epidemiology at the National Institute of Mental Health and now a professor in the department of mental hygiene at Johns Hopkins, has for several years been the lone voice warning us of this emerging crisis, which he labels an "impending pandemic."

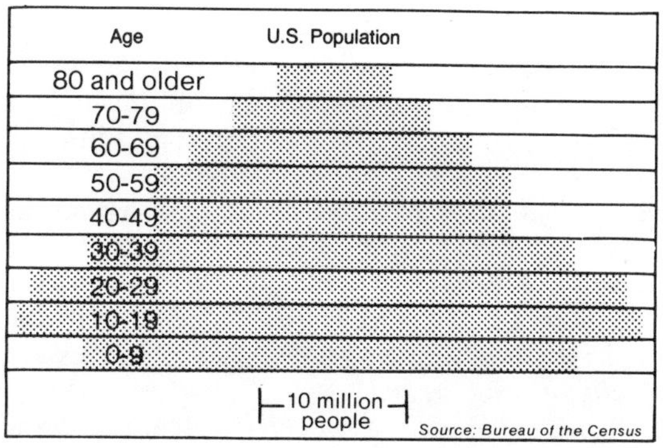

Age
U.S. Population
80 and older
70-79
60-69
50-59
40-49
30-39
20-29
10-19
0-9
10 million people
Source: Bureau of the Census

The first development that should concern us is vividly illustrated by the figure opposite. There is a huge bulge in our population curve, representing the large number of post-World War-II babies who have already begun to age into the decades where they are most likely to develop schizophrenia and other chronic or episodic psychotic conditions. This trend is occurring concomitantly with new moves to abolish state mental hospitals.

The second alarming demographic trend is the steady and continuing increase in our elderly population, which will double by the year 2020. It coincides with another development that Kramer has highlighted—the large numbers of older persons now being cared for in nursing homes. In light of the increasing awareness of how bad many nursing homes are, especially in fulfilling their residents' psychosocial needs, the scandal that could develop as our aging population and nursing home industry explode might easily eclipse any prior scandals unearthed in state hospitals.

But of more immediate concern is the dramatic increase in the number of new, young chronic patients at a time when the only remaining facilities able to provide long-term treatment and care for them are being closed. The entire mental health system now seems designed to care for the acutely ill. For these patients we do very well, with our current array of emergency services, general hospital psychiatric units, and outpatients clinics.

We also know how to care for the chronic mentally ill in the community—through community support programs that provide medication and continuing psychotherapy (aftercare) and that are linked, through case management, to other services that satisfy patients' nonmedical needs for housing, income, and vocational and social rehabilitation. But we cannot care for these patients without money and the panoply of services needed. Planners, leaders in psychiatry, and government officials simply cannot be allowed to proceed with deinstitutionalization in the absence of adequate community programs—at the very time when new, young chronic patients are emerging in unprecedented numbers.
—John A. Talbott, M.D.

Young Adult Chronic Patients: An Analytical Review of the Literature

LEONA L. BACHRACH, PH.D.
Associate Professor of Psychiatry (Sociology)
Maryland Psychiatric Research Center
Department of Psychiatry
University of Maryland School of Medicine
Baltimore, Maryland

This article analyzes the periodical and "fugitive" literature concerned with an emerging psychiatric service entity, young adult chronic patients. The increasing prominence of a young adult patient population results from the confluence of two primary forces: deinstitutionalization policies and demographic factors. The author discusses the clinical diversity and program requirements of these patients. Young adult chronic patients are best served when their uniqueness as a patient population is acknowledged and heeded and when special services for them are integrated into the total system of care, the author concludes.

■Although clinicians and administrators are becoming increasingly aware of the presence and special needs of young adult chronic mental patients, this awareness has only recently been reflected in the periodical literature. The July 1981 issue of *H&CP* contained a special section of articles dealing with this patient population (1–5). Coupled with earlier contributions by Robbins and associates (6) and Segal and associates (7,8), these articles constitute the core periodical literature that specifically focuses on young adult chronic patients as a discrete service entity. The authors address the clinical diversity and heterogeneous treatment needs of this patient population. They also discuss the barriers that obstruct young adult chronic patients' access to appropriate services.

Perhaps the characteristic that best distinguishes young adult chronic mental patients is the fact that they have generally, since the onset of their illnesses, lived in an era of deinstitutionalization (1). They are a new generation of mental patients, a generation that, in the optimism of the 1960s, was to be the beneficiary of nontraditional, noninstitutional, and nonrestrictive care (9).

What has happened to these patients? Has deinstitutionalization, the protest movement that was intended to humanize the delivery of psychiatric services (10), actually improved their lot?

The answers to these questions at the present time are not encouraging. It is becoming increasingly evident that these young patients require special programming in an era when deinstitutionalization is still conceptualized primarily as benefiting long-stay hospital patients who have been discharged. And it appears that the positive rewards of deinstitutionalization programming have largely bypassed this subgroup of the chronically mentally ill.

Some of the most informative clues regarding the existence and treatment needs of young adult chronic patients, who are roughly between the ages of 18 and 35, have come from informal spontaneous conversations at national meetings and other conferences for mental health professionals. These patients have become so popular a topic of conversation that at the April 1980 meeting of the National Council of Community Mental Health Centers in Dallas I became informally aware of their effects on service delivery in such diverse locations as Alabama, Connecticut, Massachusetts, New Hampshire, Pennsylvania, South Dakota, and Texas.

Newspaper accounts of young adult chronic patients as both victims and perpetrators of violent crimes (11–14) and as victims of service systems that typically ignore their needs (15,16) have increasingly brought members of this chronic patient subgroup to the public's attention. But young adult patients, as a separate entity, represent a topic of sufficiently recent interest that relatively little professional literature deals with issues in their care. The literature that does exist strongly reinforces informal observations and reveals that these young patients pose important problems for psychiatric service systems. The precise nature of these

Dr. Bachrach's mailing address is 11001 Wickshire Way, Rockville, Maryland 20852. This paper is based on a presentation made at "The Young Adult Chronic Patient: II," a conference sponsored by the Rockland County Community Mental Health Center and the New York State Office of Mental Health, held June 3–5, 1981, in Albany, New York. The author is indebted to the following individuals for sharing their insights regarding the care of young adult chronic patients: Robert L. DeForge, M.S., and John Pandiani, Ph.D., Montpelier, Vermont; Bert Pepper, M.D., Pomona, New York; and Robert Strange, M.D., Falls Church, Virginia.

problems is only now coming into focus, and it is apparent that demographic, clinical, and service delivery dimensions are involved (17).

This article provides an overview of issues affecting the care of young adult chronic mental patients. It is based on reviews of both the periodical literature and the "fugitive" literature—speeches, working papers, and other documents that are not readily identified through regular literature retrieval mechanisms like *Index Medicus*. It also uses, in addition to relevant articles in the popular press, the ideas of key individuals who have been directly involved in delivering services to this patient population. In this article I use the word "patient" in its broadest sense to include both actual and potential psychiatric service system enrollees.

BACKGROUND

The increasing prominence of young adult chronic mental patients results from the confluence of two primary forces: the deinstitutionalization movement that encompasses basic and far-reaching changes in patterns of service delivery to individuals with chronic mental disorders, and demographic trends in the nation's population. These factors provide a backdrop for other contributing conditions, such as the access of these young patients to street drugs, which distort their symptomatology and clinical course and complicate their treatment requirements (1981 personal communication from DeForge, 3,4,6,18). It has been reported that use of street drugs may be associated with symptomatic syndromes, relapses, and exacerbations of symptoms in individuals with severe mental disorders (19). The literature on young adult chronic patients is generally supportive of this observation.

Effects of deinstitutionalization. Deinstitutionalization, with its complicated effects on patterns of psychiatric service delivery, represents far more than the simple relocation of patients from institutional to community settings (10). It affects all components of the service delivery system and has profoundly altered service utilization patterns. Before deinstitutionalization, most individuals with chronic mental disorders were admitted to state hospitals, where they generally remained for life. They constituted an essentially static population pool that changed primarily as the result of new admissions and deaths. Providing care was relatively simple before deinstitutionalization because virtually all services for chronic patients were delivered within a single physical setting and under a single authority.

Today, however, authority for providing services to chronic mental patients is divided among many health and human service agencies in both the public and private sectors. Whereas in the past the population of chronic patients was characterized by residential stability and treatment homogeneity, today's patients are exceedingly heterogeneous in their institutional histories, and they are provided with a variety of treatment plans emanating from numerous, sometimes competing, agencies. Without the certainty of institutionalization, many patients escape the service system altogether, a situation known popularly as "falling through the cracks."

Many of today's young adult chronic mental patients represent that group of individuals who most probably would have been permanently hospitalized 25 or 30 years ago. Today, however, most chronic mental patients are no longer confined to institutions for life, and they assume increasing visibility in the psychiatric service system. A sizable number of them never enter institutions at all, not even for brief periods of care (3,4,20). Others who do enter institutions tend to stay only a short while before they are returned to the community.

Demographic factors. The salience of young adult chronic mental patients as a separate service entity is not, however, entirely an artifact of deinstitutionalization. It results instead from the interaction of changes in service delivery patterns with distinctive demographic circumstances. Since these patients are young, and since their disabilities tend to persist, there has been an accumulation of them from successive birth cohorts. This accumulation has been especially marked in recent years as postwar baby-boom babies have begun to reach maturity.

Today the 64 million babies born between 1946 and 1961 are between the ages of 21 and 36 (21). They represent nearly one-third of the nation's population. Because of their overrepresentation in the population, the absolute number of young persons at risk for developing schizophrenia and, later, other chronic mental disorders is very substantial. As predicted by Kramer (22), the coming of age of children born after World War II is now having a marked impact on the psychiatric service system.

In addition to their numerical significance, young adults in the population are, according to a report from the Bureau of the Census (23), exceedingly mobile and change their residences frequently. The highest mobility rates in the United States from 1975 to 1979 occurred among individuals in their twenties and thirties. For example, 62 per cent of persons aged 20 to 24, and 72 per cent of persons aged 25 to 29, changed residence during these years, as contrasted with 40 per cent of the total population. In all regions of the country the highest frequencies in all categories of migration, including between-state moves, occurred among individuals aged 25 to 34.

Like their nonpatient peers, many young adult chronic mental patients are highly mobile. They travel and relocate frequently within and between major cities (4,24,25) and move into and out of rural areas. The unstable residential patterns of these individuals within cities often result in their being numbered among urban "disaffiliated street people" (26). In fact, young adults are having a marked effect on the demographic composition of our cities' homeless people (24,27,28). As James A. Prevost, commissioner of mental health in New York state, says in this issue's Commentary (29), we are no longer justified in viewing vagrants as primarily elderly, impoverished "skid row" types; that stereotype has become anachronistic.

The effects of residential mobility among young adult chronic patients are also marked in rural places. In certain nonurban communities, particularly those that attract visitors and vacationers, young adult patients have imposed severe strains on the psychiatric service system. Indeed, in speaking with service providers throughout the nation, I am left with a strong impression that there are probably several large and very fluid migration streams within which young adult chronic patients move. At least one such stream affects the northeastern states and includes the rural portions of New England to the north and the metropolitan areas of New York, New Jersey, and Washington, D.C., to the south. Robert DeForge, director of alternate care programs in Washington County, Vermont, reports that the population of young adult chronic patients in his rural catchment area consists primarily of transient in-migrants who typically arrive with acute treatment, welfare, and support service requirements, including the need for money, food, and medication (1981 personal communication). Similar migration streams probably exist in other portions of the nation (30).

Another way in which nonindigenous young adult chronic patients are reported to enter rural areas is through formal admission to private psychiatric facilities. When the patients leave these facilities, often against medical advice, they remain in the surrounding communities and utilize local psychiatric resources.

Whether in rural, suburban, or urban areas, the presence of this chronic patient subgroup is increasingly reflected by psychiatric service delivery statistics. Thus, for example, Egri and Caton (31) report that the service population of the Harlem Rehabilitation Center, a special facility for chronic psychiatric patients connected with Harlem Hospital in New York City, has changed dramatically over the past 15 years. In the past most enrollees were female and over 45 years of age; today they are primarily males under 35 years of age. Bassuk (32) reports that 62 per cent of psychiatric emergency visits at a private general hospital in Boston are made by individuals 20 to 34 years old, although this group represents only 28 per cent of the general population in the catchment area. And a report from a three-county rural area in Vermont indicates that, although 25 per cent of the general population is between the ages of 20 and 34, this age group constitutes 58 per cent of those enrolled in adult community mental health programs and 52 per cent of those in substance abuse programs (33).

On the level of state services, Platman and Booker (34) report that since 1965 there has been a "striking change in the age pattern" of admissions to Maryland state psychiatric facilities, "with the age cohort 18–34 replacing 35–64 as the major admissions cohort." Similarly, Wagner (35) shows that the largest single age group of long-term chronically ill mental patients served in the Wisconsin Community Support Program consists of individuals between the ages of 18 and 35 and represents 46 per cent of the patient population.

CLINICAL DIVERSITY

Young adult chronic mental patients present a highly variable clinical picture. They constitute neither a uniform diagnostic entity nor a group with fixed and predictable symptomatology. Although they are, in some communities, predominantly male (3,4,6,7,25,31), they are by no means exclusively so. Similarly, although they are frequently diagnosed with schizophrenic disorders, they are also accorded a variety of other diagnoses, particularly that of borderline personality (2–4,36).

Indeed, the population of young adult chronic mental patients is sufficiently heterogeneous that Sheets and associates (25), in a paper published in this issue, posit three subpopulations. One consists of individuals "well ensconced in the role of patient." They are passive, apathetic, and poorly motivated persons who, even in remission, exhibit extreme dependency on the psychiatric service system. Another category contains individuals who are highly motivated and who function well in remission but are nonetheless "seriously disabled by their disorders." They are often isolated individuals with limited social supports and little hope of lasting success despite their aspirations.

Sheets and associates' other category conforms most closely to the young adult chronic patients portrayed in most of the literature. The individuals in this group are described as aggressive and basically noncompliant persons who have low tolerance for frustration and whose "low frustration tolerance and impulsive behaviors frequently result in encounters with the law" (25). These are the individuals who are frequently mobile—within a single psychiatric service system ("revolving door" patients), within their areas of residence, between cities, and between states. Schwartz and Goldfinger (4) point out that, although these individuals have a "wide range of ego deficits," such as defects in impulse control and affective modulation, the "extent to which these defects dominate the clinical picture, and the degree to which they incapacitate the patient, appears widely variable." Steyn (37) refers to these patients as individuals who "have not entered adulthood despite their years." Pepper and associates (3) share this developmental view and assert that these patients "are stuck in the transition from childhood dependency to adult independence."

IMPACT ON THE SERVICE SYSTEM

If young adult chronic mental patients are so diverse that they defy description through a single clinical profile, by what logic are they grouped together as a separate service entity? The answer to this question lies in their collective impact on the psychiatric service system. Pepper and associates (3) write that these patients share two "overarching characteristics"—severe deficits in social functioning and a "tendency to use mental health services inappropriately, in ways that drain the time and energy of clinicians yet do not conform to viable treatment plans."

Thus, wherever they are found, and whatever their specific difficulties may be, the existence of young adult chronic patients is typically associated with severe system stress. This situation is at least partially explained by the widespread absence of community supports for these patients. Young adult chronic patients generally alienate family, friends, and other crisis resources, and the psychiatric service system must assume a major support role during the recurrent crises in their lives (4).

Young adult chronic mental patients are pervasive users of the psychiatric service system; they tend to utilize state psychiatric facilities, community mental health centers, private psychiatric hospitals, general hospitals, and a variety of outpatient facilities (3,4,25,31,34–41). Lamb (42,43) reports that in California young adult chronic patients are heavily represented in the populations of locked skilled nursing facilities that are community-based and, to a lesser extent, of board-and-care homes.

In some parts of the country these patients are found in single-room-occupancy hotels (SROs). The New York State Department of Social Services (44) reports that nearly a third of Manhattan's westside SRO residents, a majority of whom exhibit varying degrees of psychopathology (45), are under the age of 35. Young adult chronic patients in SROs are reported to have various special program needs (46).

Despite their enrollment in a wide variety of psychiatric and social services, at any given time a substantial portion of young adult chronic patients are *not* enrolled in psychiatric facilities and are essentially unserved by the psychiatric service system. As indicated previously, growing numbers of them have been documented as street people, particularly in California and New York (7,8,27,29,30). Yet they constitute a distinct subgroup even within this larger disaffiliated population. Segal and Baumohl (8) refer to them as "space cases," who are "judged by other street people to be delusionary, unpredictable, and unreliable—in the lexicon of the street, 'burned out,' 'fried,' or 'spaced.' "

Those young adult chronic patients who use psychiatric services generally do so in a revolving-door manner and move frequently from one facility to another. Many are also involved intermittently with the criminal justice system (1,3,7,8,11,29). Robbins and associates describe these patients as being in a "state of disequilibrium because they cannot adapt to the community and cannot remain in the hospital." Often, if they are admitted to hospitals, "they refuse to remain more than a short time, either requesting a discharge or eloping. When in the community they do not participate for long, if at all, in therapeutic programs" (6).

In some communities these patients become general hospital emergency room regulars (4,32,38,47,48). Unfortunately, however, the "classic models of emergency intervention are grossly inappropriate to their needs" (4). Their referral out of the emergency room to other facilities tends to be exceedingly problematic, because they are difficult to engage in treatment and appear to have no established niche in the psychiatric service system.

Young adult chronic patients who use psychiatric services generally do so in a revolving-door manner and move frequently from one facility to another. Many are involved with the criminal justice system.

In short, young adult chronic mental patients are ubiquitous and, according to many service providers, very troublesome. They are properly described as chronic patients in that they conform to at least three important criteria of chronicity as described by Peele and Palmer (49): they have substantial deficits in functioning; they exhibit continued dependency in their life styles; and they show evidence of indefinite need for psychiatric and social support services.

Many agencies frankly do not know quite what to do with these young people. Harris and Bergman (40) at St. Elizabeths Hospital in Washington, D.C., write, "After several rounds of bouncing between hospital and community, no one expects these patients to change. They are treated perfunctorily . . . by a staff that is too discouraged to do more than go through the motions."

This description from an inner-city service setting is paralleled by a similar picture in a rural portion of the nation. DeForge (1981 personal communication) indicates that in rural Vermont the young adult chronic patient population consists primarily of individuals who "will confound all your treatment efforts, who will take your emergency workers and your other treatment people and run them in circles for many hours and many days, so that the staff reaction to them is basically a lot of anger and frustration."

Nor are suburban communities immune. Steyn (37), a psychiatrist at an intermediate-stay state psychiatric facility in the suburbs of Washington, D.C., compares the behavior of young adult chronic patients to that of neglected children "who want what they want when they want it, if they know what they want, and throw the adult equivalent of temper tantrums when they don't get it."

There is little question that these young patients tend to fall squarely within the category of individuals described by Chrzanowski (50) as "problem patients," who are socially unresponsive, hostile, and acting-out individuals with a "high degree of therapeutic immunity." Similarly, they conform to Neill's (41) description of "difficult patients"—demanding and manipulative individuals whose "presence engenders strong negative feelings—anger, fear, helplessness among members of the treatment staff." These patients' patterns of social interaction tend to be highly affect-laden, so that in therapeutic situations they are often characterized by "instantaneous transference" (50). In turn, they are apt to generate serious countertransference reactions in their therapists (DeForge, 1981 personal communication).

PROGRAM REQUIREMENTS

A series of eight program principles shared by successful model programs for the chronically mentally ill have been identified in the literature (51). These principles appear to hold for young chronic patients as well as for other subgroups of the chronically mentally ill (52,53). According to these principles, programs that work for chronic mental patients assign top priority to the care of the most severely impaired patients and thereby eliminate their need to compete for services; enable patients to gain access to a full range of comprehensive services; are realistically linked to other agencies and resources that assist patients; are characterized by personally designed and highly individualized services; emphasize the need for specially trained staff who are aware of the unique needs of the chronically mentally ill; show flexibility in their formats so that they may change readily in response to the changing needs of their enrollees; are tied in some manner to a complement of hospital beds; and are relevant to and compatible with the culture base in the particular communities where they are located.

Because these program principles generally form a least common denominator for program design for the chronically mentally ill (51), they may be used to assess the program requirements of particular chronic patient populations. It is clear from the literature, however, that programs in which young adult chronic patients are enrolled are, for the most part, lacking in the application of these principles. Even a cursory review reveals a basic lack of concordance between these principles and actual efforts to provide services for this target group.

The following discussion documents fundamental disparities between what is known and what is done in the provision of services to young adult chronic patients. Although a fairly well-developed technology exists for their care, the means for applying that technology often lag. In part the problem is conceptual—the failure of service planners and providers to recognize the unique position of these patients. The problem is also, to a considerable extent, attitudinal. These young patients are not only stigmatized in the public view but are also difficult patients whom staff either cannot or will not serve effectively.

Comprehensive services. There is a strong emphasis in the literature on the need for a full range of comprehensive services—including psychiatric, medical, rehabilitative, vocational, social, and residential services—for young adult chronic patients (31,39,40,46,54). Adequate residential services appear, for many writers, to be the sine qua non of comprehensive services and the foundation upon which the comprehensive service structure must be built. This is particularly true in the literature that deals with the special needs of young adult patients who are currently homeless (7,8,24,28,55–57).

The need for comprehensive services for young adult chronic patients is so basic that an approach that integrates programs for these patients into the larger service system is required. The imaginative programs available to young adult patients in Rockland County, New York, (3,18,54) exemplify the advantages of systems planning and provide a striking example of what can be accomplished when the special needs of these patients have been acknowledged.

Resource linkage. The literature reports that because services for young adult patients are typically fragmented and planned under different auspices, special efforts for coordinating and integrating programs must be undertaken. A New York State report specifically calls for innovative interagency linkages in services for individuals living in SROs (46), and the literature contains similar pleas for patients in other residential settings.

One specific example of an effectively linked program reported in the *New York Times* (56) describes a residential facility in lower Manhattan. Operated by Franciscan friars, the facility provides residents with room and board and arranges the delivery of social, recreational, prevocational, psychiatric, and medical services, including semiweekly visits from physicians at Bellevue Hospital. Resources like this one are rare, however, and stand out primarily as examples of what might be accomplished under ideal circumstances.

Some of the literature stresses case management as an effective, even an essential, means for linking and integrating services for young adult chronic patients (3,40,54). The discussion that follows will demonstrate, however, that case management and other vital services that help assure patients' continuity of care are, at times, systematically denied to young adult patients.

Individualized treatment. Kirshner and Ryglewicz (54) observe that for young adult chronic patients "there must be a matrix of services to deal with individual needs and the varying intensity of those needs; for times when the patient is in partial remission and able to work on his problems, yet feeling he doesn't need to; and for times when he or she is in crisis." Thus it is essential that services for these patients be highly individualized. This is true for psychiatric services, as well as rehabilitative and social services. Sheets and associates (25) observe that certain young adult patients need and will accept traditional sheltered workshop arrangements, while others require "more creative vocational programs." Similarly, some of these patients may benefit from neighborhood psychosocial club arrangements, while others are better suited to socialization opportunities in a variety of settings, including homes, restaurants, and pubs. Still other patients may profit most from youth-oriented drop-in centers (25).

Specially trained staff. In a general discussion of difficult patients Groves (58) makes the point that, "admitted or not," these individuals tend to "kindle aversion, fear, despair, or even downright malice in their doctors. Emotional reactions to patients cannot simply be wished away, nor is it good medicine to pretend that they do not exist." The literature endorses Groves' position with specific reference to young adult chronic patients. Schwartz and Goldfinger (4) write that as these patients "alternately demand and reject care, as they alternate between dependency, manipulation, withdrawal, anger, depression, and other interactive styles and emotional states, even the most tolerant and resourceful clinician is likely to experience increasing anger, bitterness, frustration, and helplessness. These responses, in turn, can lead to even more inappropriate treatment decisions, which are not in anyone's long-term interests but only serve to remove the patient, temporarily, from the responsibility of a given caretaker."

Thus it is not surprising that much of the literature stresses the need for specially trained staff who are prepared to deal with the unique needs of these young patients (40,47,59). Harris and Bergman (40) go so far as to call for a "new breed of mental health professionals who can bridge the gap between the hospital and community" and who can work "flexibly and integratively" in diverse service settings.

Part of the specialized training of staff should, ideally, deal with the burnout that they inevitably will experience. Egri (39) suggests that staff who deal daily with chronic patients will benefit from seminars focusing on the management of burnout: "An opportunity to be heard, appreciated, supported, and stimulated to contribute new ideas by peers and supervisors recharges the energies so constantly drained by demands of a very needy patient population."

Flexible programs. The need for great flexibility in program design is widely endorsed in the literature. Some sources emphasize the need for flexibility in specific program areas. Thus, for example, Pauldine (60) advocates the development of intensive and flexible follow-up mechanisms for the period immediately after discharge from a psychiatric facility, a time when young adult patients are most apt to be lost to the mental health system. Similarly, Ryglewicz (61) discusses the need for flexibility in communicating with patients' families. Because their family situations are so varied, no single format of family involvement or family therapy can be used universally. Most of the literature encourages flexibility in all program initiatives so that the diverse needs of this heterogeneous patient group, and their changing patterns of residence, can be accommodated.

Hospital beds. One may infer from the literature that young adult chronic patients often do not, or cannot, use existing inpatient services optimally (4,6,7). They are likely to leave hospitals, often against medical advice, before they can reap maximum benefit from the hospital experience. This does not mean that the notion of hospital beds or inpatient care for the young adult chronic patient population should be abandoned altogether and that these individuals should not, under any circumstances, be hospitalized. It does mean that, for those times when inpatient care is necessary, planning should be directed toward placing the patient in the most therapeutic environment (62).

It is reported that, for some young adult chronic patients, episodes of state hospital care are most therapeutic, provided that these facilities can adapt their programs to the special and flexible needs of this patient group (6,40). For others in this special population, however, it seems more therapeutic to provide care in nontraditional and noninstitutional settings that are close to patients' homes. Sometimes it is possible to use hospital bed equivalents. Lamb (43), for example, describes the use of locked skilled nursing facilities with highly structured environments as one possible alternative to hospitalization that provides inpatient care without necessitating removal of patients from their home communities. This alternative is particularly viable for those patients who require a high degree of structure. For other members of the young adult patient group, particularly those with borderline personality diagnoses, inhospital treatment on short-term open general hospital units, with moderately structured environments, may be indicated (63).

What is important is that the range of available inpatient facilities, or their nursing home or other functional equivalents, be sufficiently diverse to meet the heterogeneous needs of the full range of young adult chronic patients.

Cultural relevance. One of the most important program principles to honor in planning services for young adult chronic patients is that of cultural relevance and compatibility. Egri (39) captures the essence of this principle in her description of the Harlem Rehabilitation Center, which is physically separated from the rest of Harlem Hospital by seven city blocks: "The very fact of separation enhances . . . perception [of the Center] as a community facility by patients, diminishing their sense of 'patienthood' and dependence, thus reinforcing the passage of independence and autonomy so essential to successful rehabilitation. In the neighborhood the Center is known as 'the school.' "

While the physical separation of facilities for young adult chronic patients is not necessarily a practicable or desirable step to follow in all programs, Egri's statement reflects a recurrent theme in the literature—the cultural irrelevance of many traditional mental health programs to the needs of young adult chronic patients. This deficit is noted both for patients enrolled in hospital-based programs (25,31,40) and, more particularly, for those who are among the population of vagrant street people (8,27,55).

For the latter subgroup of young adult chronic patients, it is important that programs be planned with an appreciation of the uniqueness of street culture, which tends to differ materially from the cultural exposures of most mental health workers. Some of the nuances of street culture include special survival skills, a special language, and unique sources of prestige (27). Accordingly, Segal and Baumohl (8) write that, in order to engage California's young adult vagrant patient population in treatment, lengthy paperwork procedures and formal treatment settings should be avoided. They assert that coffee houses and community "living rooms" work most effectively as treatment settings, because they are "typically open to anyone and are unencumbered by intake and assessment protocols that ritually confirm clienthood and are perceived [by patients] as threats or create formality or social distance."

Top priority. For the most part, young adult chronic mental patients have great difficulty in fitting into established program settings. They certainly require the kind of top priority assignment in service delivery that would exempt them from competing for services, in accord with the first model program planning principle, because they have some very special problems in gaining access to the service system. They are quintessentially patients who are difficult to treat and who are apt to be rejected wherever they are found.

Psychiatric service systems, without some alterations, are not designed for young adult chronic mental patients, who have been described as "career" mental patients destined to become "the most difficult mental patients of the 1980's" (8). These patients will probably continue to drift in and out of the psychiatric service system and to impose great stresses on it unless high priority is placed on developing specialized programs, with highly individualized treatment interventions, for their care.

It is clear, too, that unless some special effort is made to integrate the needs of these patients into the greater system of psychiatric services, as it has been in Rockland County, New York, young adult chronic patients will be overlooked and rejected. Even with the exemplary systems approach that has been adopted in Rockland County, there are several limiting external systems constraints, such as those imposed by skewed eligibility requirements for state Community Support System (CSS) services. This situation, ironically, rewards institutionalization instead of urging optimal and relevant community-based care.

Kirshner and Ryglewicz (54), for example, report that although case management services have proved extremely beneficial to young adult chronic patients, state-supported case management is reserved for patients who have had at least six consecutive months of psychiatric hospitalization, who have had at least three discrete psychiatric hospitalizations of at least ten days each, or who have had three months of cumulative psychiatric hospitalization in the two years preceding application for services (38). The result is that as many as 55 per cent of young adult chronic patients in Rockland County are barred from state-supported case management services (54). It is not surprising that a New York state case management evaluation report has suggested redrawing CSS eligibility guidelines so that patient need and not previous hospitalization may become the basic criterion (64).

It is essential that entitlements and benefits for these patients not be tied in any way to their having undergone periods of care inside hospitals if the basic goal of deinstitutionalization—humanizing mental health services by providing them primarily in community-based settings close to home (10)—is to be fulfilled. Yet this is precisely the paradox that faces many young adult chronic patients.

PLANNING FOR THE FUTURE

When yardsticks of effective program design are used to assess services for young adult chronic patients, it becomes evident that there are serious impediments to service delivery for this target population. The disjunction between the process of deinstitutionalization and the philosophy that underlies it (10) is glaringly evident with respect to this patient group. The disjunction is apparent in the gross irrelevance of many interventions to the needs of young adult chronic patients. And it is manifested in such disparities as giving lip service to community-based programs while impeding patients' access to entitlements that would enable them to remain in the community. Not only is their access to CSS eligibility limited in some jurisdictions, but they are also reported to have difficulties with other entitlements like Supplemental Security Income benefits (7,8).

In general, existing treatment settings are not optimally geared toward young adult chronic mental patients, even when active efforts on behalf of the chronically mentally ill have been undertaken. Primary emphasis in deinstitutionalization programming has traditionally been, and continues to be, on aftercare for discharged institutional residents instead of on providing services to preclude the necessity for institutionalization in the first place. Although the never-hospitalized are as much products of deinstitutionalization policies and practices as are state hospital dischargees (10), many, probably most, planned deinstitutionalization efforts serve a population that is already distinguished by the syndrome Goffman (65) termed "institutionalism."

More research on the program needs of young adult chronic patients is strongly indicated. Schwartz and Goldfinger (4) write that "further empirical research and analysis are needed to provide a more precise and comprehensive picture of the characteristics of this emerging subgroup, of their interactions with a variety of community mental health services, and of the consequences of these interactions." Indeed, very little research has been done on the outcomes of selected treatment interventions. Studies such as that by Caton (1), which shows high rates of criminal activity, arrest, and suicide among inner-city, previously hospitalized, young adult patients diagnosed as being schizophrenic, should certainly be expanded and replicated.

It is important, too, that design biases affecting the

quality of research be kept to a minimum. Baxter and Hopper (27) have found, for example, that the life circumstances of their study population of homeless adults—including many young adult chronic patients—in New York City do not readily lend themselves to study by "conventional research methods," such as controlled or quantitative study designs. However, by applying participant observation techniques, these investigators have amassed critical information about the aspirations, adaptations, and problems of their study population.

Finally, it is important to remember as we plan for the care of young adult chronic mental patients that they are part of an aging population. As they grow older, their service needs will change. At some time in the future they will become a geriatric population for which the psychiatric service system must be prepared.

In the future, as today, this special target population will best be served if its uniqueness is appreciated and heeded. Without special planning, these young adult patients will probably, at best, become the "new long-stay" institutional population (10) of tomorrow, or, at worst, will receive no psychiatric services at all. Their right to specialized care—to planning that is adapted to their special needs and not simply incidental to aftercare for institutional dischargees—must be firmly established.■

REFERENCES

1) Caton CLM: The new chronic patient and the system of community care. Hospital & Community Psychiatry 32:475–478, 1981

2) Green RS, Koprowski PF: The chronic patient with a nonpsychotic diagnosis. Hospital & Community Psychiatry 32:479–481, 1981

3) Pepper B, Kirshner MC, Ryglewicz H: The young adult chronic patient: overview of a population. Hospital & Community Psychiatry 32:463–469, 1981

4) Schwartz SR, Goldfinger SM: The new chronic patient: clinical characteristics of an emerging subgroup. Hospital & Community Psychiatry 32:470–474, 1981

5) Talbott JA: The emerging crisis in chronic care. Hospital & Community Psychiatry 32:447, 1981

6) Robbins E, Stern M, Robbins L, et al: Unwelcome patients: where can they find asylum? Hospital & Community Psychiatry 29:44–46, 1978

7) Segal SP, Baumohl J, Johnson E: Falling through the cracks: mental disorder and social margin in a young vagrant population. Social Problems 24:387–400, 1977

8) Segal SP, Baumohl J: Engaging the disengaged: proposals on madness and vagrancy. Social Work 25:358–365, 1980

9) Kennedy JF: Message From the President of the United States Relative to Mental Illness and Mental Retardation, House of Representatives Document 58, February 5, 1963

10) Bachrach LL: A conceptual approach to deinstitutionalization. Hospital & Community Psychiatry 29:573–578, 1978

11) Basler B: Assault on officer and a drifter's lack of treatment. New York Times, May 12, 1981, p A1

12) Buder L: Man with razor seized in slashings of vagrants. New York Times, July 7, 1981, p A1

13) Herman R: Funds asked for sites to contain violent patients. New York Times, March 8, 1981, p 43

14) McFadden RD: A violent RI man dies while being subdued. New York Times, Aug 2, 1981, p 30

15) Cohn R: Outside: one man, mentally ill and trapped. Philadelphia Inquirer, May 1, 1978, p B1

16) Robinson E, Pearson R: Shelters for homeless are filled to capacity during bitter weather. Washington Post, Dec 27, 1980, p C1

17) Wykert J: Young chronic patient called growing concern. Psychiatric News, June 5, 1981, p 12

18) Pepper B, Ryglewicz H: An uninstitutionalized generation: psychiatrically disabled young people in the community. Presented at the Conference on the Young Adult Chronic Patient II, Albany, NY, June 3–5, 1981

19) Pearlson GD: Psychiatric and medical syndromes associated with phencyclidine (PCP) abuse. Johns Hopkins Medical Journal 148:25–33, 1981

20) Cancro focuses on functioning of schizophrenic youths. Psychiatric News, March 6, 1981, p 50

21) Beck M, Witherspoon D, Foote D, et al: The baby boomers come of age. Newsweek, March 30, 1981, pp 34–37

22) Kramer M: Psychiatric Services and the Changing Institutional Scene, 1950–1985. Rockville, Md, National Institute of Mental Health, 1977

23) US Bureau of the Census: Geographical Mobility: March 1975 to March 1979. Washington, DC, US Government Printing Office, 1980

24) Carmody D: New York is facing "crisis" on vagrants. New York Times, June 28, 1981, p 1

25) Sheets JL, Prevost J, Reihman J: Young adult chronic patients: three hypothesized subgroups. Hospital & Community Psychiatry. 33:197–203, 1982

26) New York State Office of Mental Health: New York State's versus New York City's Record in Mental Health and Social Services. Albany, NY, Dec 29, 1980

27) Baxter E, Hopper K: Private Lives/Public Spaces: Homeless Adults on the Streets of New York City. New York Community Service Society, 1981

28) Bird D: A quiet retreat for city's homeless. New York Times, June 9, 1981, p B1

29) Prevost JA: Youthful chronicity: paradox of the 80s. Hospital & Community Psychiatry 33:173, 1982

30) Timnick L: The new drifters: society's costly and dangerous burden. Los Angeles Times, July 20, 1981, p 13

31) Egri G, Caton CL: Serving the young adult chronic patient in the 1980s: challenge to the general hospital. Presented at the meeting of the American Association for General Hospital Psychiatry, San Diego, Calif, Sept 13, 1981

32) Bassuk EL: The impact of deinstitutionalization on the general hospital psychiatric emergency ward. Hospital & Community Psychiatry 31:623–627, 1980

33) Pandiani J, Butterfield C: Client profile and condition on termination of clients served by community mental health centers in central Vermont. Montpelier, Vt, Washington County Mental Health Services, 1980

34) Platman SR, Booker TC: The Changing Nature of the State Mental Hospital System. Baltimore, Maryland Department of Health and Mental Hygiene, 1981

35) Wagner BA: Progress Report: Community Support Programs for the Long-Term Mentally Ill in Wisconsin. Madison, Wis, Wisconsin Bureau of Mental Health, 1981

36) Lehmann JB: Mental Health Follow-Up Care Updated. Elgin, Ill, Elgin Mental Health Center, 1979

37) Steyn RW: Tomorrow's patients: our changing patient population. Advance, summer-fall 1981, pp 15–17

38) Caton CL: New York City Community Support Systems Monitoring and Evaluation Project. New York, New York State Psychiatric Institute, 1981

39) Egri G: A general hospital model, in The Chronic Mentally Ill: Treatment, Programs, Systems. Edited by Talbott JA. New York, Human Sciences Press, 1981

40) Harris M, Bergman H: Coordination of inpatient hospitalization and community support programs: an integrated systems approach. Washington, DC, St Elizabeths Hospital, 1979

41) Neill JR: The difficult patient: identification and response. Journal of Clinical Psychiatry 40: 209–212, 1979

42) Lamb HR: The new asylums in the community. Archives of General Psychiatry 36:129–134, 1979

43) Lamb HR: Structure: the neglected ingredient of community

treatment. Archives of General Psychiatry 37:1224–1228, 1980
44) Survey of the Needs and Problems of Single Room Occupancy Hotel Residents on the Upper West Side of Manhattan, New York City: Final Report of the SRO Project. Albany, NY, New York State Department of Social Services, 1980
45) Sokolovsky J, Cohen C, Berger D, et al: Ex-mental patients in a Manhattan SRO hotel. Human Organization 37:5–15, 1978
46) Epple WA, Steadman HJ: A Survey of Services for SRO Residents in Manhattan. Albany, NY, New York State Office of Mental Health Bureau of Special Projects Research, 1979
47) Bassuk E, Gerson S: Chronic crisis patients: a discrete clinical group. American Journal of Psychiatry 137:1513–1517, 1980
48) Gerson S, Bassuk E: Psychiatric emergencies: an overview. American Journal of Psychiatry 137:1–11, 1980
49) Peele R, Palmer RR: Patient rights and patient chronicity. Journal of Psychiatry and Law, spring 1980, pp 59–71
50) Chrzanowski G: Problem patients or troublemakers? Dynamic and therapeutic considerations. American Journal of Psychotherapy 34:26–38, 1980
51) Bachrach LL: Overview: model programs for chronic mental patients. American Journal of Psychiatry 137:1023–1031, 1980
52) Mosher LR, Menn AZ: Community residential treatment for schizophrenia: two-year follow-up. Hospital & Community Psychiatry 29:715–723, 1978
53) Mosher LR, Menn AZ: Lowered barriers in the community: the Soteria model, in Alternatives to Mental Hospital Treatment. Edited by Stein LI, Test MA. New York, Plenum, 1978
54) Kirshner MC, Ryglewicz H: The psychiatrically disabled young adult patient: the Rockland County Community Mental Health Center's programmatic response. Presented at the Conference on the Young Adult Chronic Patient II, Albany, NY, June 3–5, 1981
55) Bird D: Help is urged for 36,000 homeless in city's streets. New York Times, March 8, 1981, p 1
56) Bird D: Wanderers find shelter and a new life. New York Times, April 21, 1981, p B6
57) Carmody D: Proposed referral center for homeless disturbs west side neighborhood. New York Times, May 25, 1981, p B5
58) Groves JE: Taking care of the hateful patient. New England Journal of Medicine 298:883–887, 1978
59) Ward R: A psychiatrist's plea: help young adults. Albany Knickerbocker News, June 4, 1981, p 3A
60) Pauldine D: Introduction: case conference and discharge planning. Presented at the Conference on the Young Adult Chronic Patient II, Albany, NY, June 3–5, 1981
61) Ryglewicz H: Working with the family of the psychiatrically disabled young adult. Presented at the Conference on the Young Adult Chronic Patient II, Albany, NY, June 3–5, 1981
62) Bachrach LL: Is the least restrictive environment always the best? Sociological and semantic implications. Hospital & Community Psychiatry 31:97–103, 1980
63) Kibel HD: The rationale for the use of group psychotherapy for borderline patients on a short-term unit. International Journal of Group Psychotherapy 28:339–358, 1978
64) Baker F, Intagliata J, Kirshstein R: Case Management Evaluation Phase One Final Report. Albany, NY, New York State Office of Mental Health, 1980
65) Goffman E: Asylums: Essays on the Social Situation of Mental Patients and Other Inmates. Garden City, NY, Anchor Books, 1961

Young Adult Chronic Patients: Three Hypothesized Subgroups

JOHN L. SHEETS, M.S.W., M.P.H.
Director of Rehabilitation Services
Hutchings Psychiatric Center
Syracuse, New York

JAMES A. PREVOST, M.D.
Commissioner
New York State Office of Mental Health
Albany, New York

JACQUELINE REIHMAN, PH.D.
Director of Program Evaluation
Hutchings Psychiatric Center
Syracuse, New York

Shortly after the 1963 passage of the Community Mental Health Centers Act, New York State launched the construction of four new psychiatric centers, including the Richard H. Hutchings Psychiatric Center in Syracuse. The Hutchings acute care crisis stabilization model was intended to significantly diminish the phenomenon of chronic psychiatric disability. After a decade of operation, however, the Hutchings Center must deal with a caseload of young and chronically disabled individuals who are contributing to the build-up both in the hospital and in the community of the new long-stay patient. The idiosyncratic needs of this chronic group must be defined so that prescriptive programs can be built to meet their needs. The Hutchings Center's original goal of returning patients to and serving them in the community remains the same, but the process of treatment, rehabilitation, and long-term community support must change.

■In 1965 New York state launched a mental health facilities construction program. The purpose of this program was to merge new concepts in architectural design, size, and location with the innovative philosophies of community mental health programming. As a

Dr. Prevost is also professor of psychiatry and Mr. Sheets and Dr. Reihman are assistant professors of psychiatry at the State University of New York Upstate Medical Center in Syracuse. Mr. Sheets' address is Hutchings Psychiatric Center, Box 27, University Station, Syracuse, New York 13210. This paper is based on a presentation at conferences on "The Young Adult Chronic Patient: Clinical and Programmatic Issues" sponsored by the Rockland County Community Mental Health Center and the New York State Office of Mental Health, November 20–21, 1980, in Suffern, New York, and June 3–5, 1981, in Albany, New York. The authors thank the staff of the Hutchings Psychiatric Center's rehabilitation and program evaluation departments for contributing to the development and analysis of data.

result, four new urban-based psychiatric centers, including the Richard H. Hutchings Psychiatric Center in Syracuse, opened during the early 1970s.

Hutchings began by assuming service responsibility for Onondaga County, which currently has a metropolitan population of 463,000. Since that time, the facility has expanded its catchment area to include four rural counties and now serves a population of 770,000. Today the system serves children, adults, and geriatric patients and consists of 150 inpatient beds, day treatment and case management programs, a network of neighborhood-based outpatient clinics, a comprehensive rehabilitation program, and access to voluntary agency, vocational rehabilitation, psychosocial club, and alternative housing programs. Currently the average daily census at Hutchings is 1,500 patients; of these, only 10 per cent occupy inpatient beds.

From its inception Hutchings differed from older state institutions because it did not have an aged and chronically institutionalized population to serve. It was designed to embrace the community mental health ideology and focus new programs on relatively young patients who were entering the mental health system for the first time.

Imbued with optimism, Hutchings set out to stabilize patients through the short-term crisis-oriented services of an acute-care model. The Hutchings staff intended not only to treat serious mental disorder but to prevent the scars of chronicity so widely associated with long-term hospital care. The ultimate symbol of this treatment optimism was that Hutchings had no back-up hospital to which it could transfer patients who did not respond to or who were not well served by an acute treatment model. Returning patients to community placements was Hutchings' only transfer option.

Because of its programs, treatment philosophy, and patient characteristics, the experience of Hutchings closely resembles that reported for certain community mental health centers (1), unitized state hospitals (2), and general hospital psychiatric programs (3). Thus the problems and experiences of the Hutchings staff may reflect a trend that will probably influence most of the nation's mental health service providers.

THE PROBLEM SITUATION

Hutchings has witnessed continuous growth and change during the past decade. The most profound change occurred during 1980, when Hutchings recorded an unprecedented increase in the number of persons seeking evaluation and admission to service. While 3,000 persons requested service in 1979, the 1980 total of 3,600 persons represents an annual increase of 20 per cent. This obviously poses significant problems to an acute care center with 19 beds per 100,000 population and no option for transfer except to community placement. Increased admissions and occupancy rates will result in a build-up of long-stay patients on the inpatient units and fewer available acute care beds.

POSSIBLE CAUSES

There are many hypotheses that could be offered to account for this increase in evaluations and admissions. The first hypothesis derives from the work of Kramer (4), who forecast an absolute nationwide increase through 1985 in the number of persons with serious mental disorder. This epidemiologic argument is grounded in the relative increase in the total population of those age groups that typically exhibit the initial onset of schizophrenia and other serious mental disorder, that is, individuals aged 15 to 44.

The second hypothesis, and the one that appears most responsible for the current bed crisis, concerns the build-up of new long-stay inpatients. This is particularly true of those young adults who are difficult to place in community settings because of a history of arson or assault, or a diagnosis of mental retardation, or because they are being held under criminal proceedings. It is also true of older patients who need skilled nursing, which is often extremely difficult to arrange, or other health-related care. Currently, for example, more than 35 per cent of all inpatients at Hutchings have been there for 90 days or more, and 10 per cent have been there for more than a year. Although lengths of stay of this duration are not unusual in a traditional state hospital or long-term-care facility, they create serious bed shortages in an acute care center.

Another hypothesis for this rising service pressure is that the community mental health model, designed to eliminate or at least mitigate chronic psychiatric disability, has not succeeded. In fact, serious and persistent psychiatric disorders are pervasive, demanding our attention and shaping still another era of mental health system change.

Nowhere is this change in service demands more compelling than in the treatment of young adults who are entering the system with alarming regularity and who, as Pepper (5) suggests, "confound our efforts to treat them by conventional means."

SUGGESTED SOLUTIONS

The challenge presented by this service-demand crisis suggests the need to make important organizational and

In 1980 Hutchings had an unprecedented increase in the number of persons seeking evaluation and admission. . . . This poses significant problems to an acute care center with 19 beds per 100,000 and no option for transfer except community placement.

clinical changes. Perhaps the most urgent need is to design service interventions for the emerging young adult chronic population that will be prescriptive and hence more effective. In the next decade young adult chronic patients will become the single largest population group requiring services from mental health systems; thus it is essential to establish baseline information regarding their salient features. Before services can be effectively developed, it is necessary to define who and how many constitute the young adult chronic population, what their service needs are, and what impact they are having on the current service system.

DEFINING AND COUNTING

At Hutchings this identification phase has already begun. Using a conceptual framework developed by Minkoff (6), we found that chronicity may be defined in any of three ways: by diagnosis, which typically includes organic conditions, schizophrenia, the major affective disorders, and some personality disorders; by duration of stay, usually defined as one year or more of hospitalization; and by disability, usually defined as an impairment of role performance or daily living skills. Goldman and associates (7) and Wing (8) have also reported that chronicity of long-term patients maintained in the community, at least in terms of functional disability, may also be inferred from the services they use, for example, sheltered workshops, supervised residences, and day programs. We constructed indicators for each of these chronicity criteria and applied them to 2,361 individuals of all ages who were served by the facility in 1979. We judged 1,232, or 52 per cent, of all patients to be chronic by a combination of diagnosis, duration of stay, and disability criteria.

Since the single largest age group served by Hutchings is that of the young adult (18 to 34 years old), we hypothesized that a significant proportion of those regarded as chronic had not been in the system long enough to have been regarded as chronic according to the more traditional diagnosis or duration-of-stay criteria. This hypothesis was supported when we eliminated both diagnosis and history of hospitalization and found that 966, or 41 per cent, of Hutchings' 1979 population could be described as chronic by functional disability alone. Further, of those 966 persons judged chronic on the basis of functional disability, 369, or 36 per cent, were between the ages of 18 and 34.

PATIENT CHARACTERISTICS

To clarify the clinical and demographic characteristics of the young adult patients at Hutchings, we developed a statistical description of the average young adult patient in 1979 and compared it with similar everyman-everywoman profiles for older chronic patients. According to this composite, the young chronically disabled adult at Hutchings is a single white male, age 27, who lives in the city of Syracuse as opposed to the suburbs. He was first admitted to Hutchings on an involuntary status when he was 22 years old and received a diagnosis of schizophrenia. Since then he has been hospitalized slightly less than once a year. Each hospitalization is usually a short stay averaging less than 30 days. Since his first inpatient admission three years ago he has been admitted and/or transferred five times to inpatient, outpatient, and day-treatment services. During 1979 he received both inpatient and outpatient services and used either a supervised residence or a supervised day program. As of January 1980, he was still being actively followed by the Hutchings service.

If we compare the young adult chronic patient with the middle-aged chronic patient at Hutchings, we find that the profiles are similar except that the middle-aged patient is a 49-year-old woman who entered the system for the first time when she was 43 and since that time has been hospitalized slightly less than once every two years. In 1979 she used only outpatient services and, like her young adult counterpart, she was still active in the system as of July 1980.

TABLE 1 Community functioning problems of Hutchings patients[1]

	Per cent reporting problems	
Community functioning domain	18 to 35 years	36+ years
Physical disabilities	45%	70%
Personal hygiene	31%	35%
Psychiatric symptoms	47%	20%
Daily living skills	66%	53%
Behavior problems	35%	8%
Social isolation	73%	59%
Alcohol, drug abuse	25%	11%

[1] Based on information developed by the New York State Office of Mental Health's Bureau of Program Evaluation, 44 Holland Avenue, Albany, New York.

COMMUNITY FUNCTIONING

We gathered data on the community functioning of chronic patients who were 36 or older and compared these findings with data on the community functioning of young adult chronic patients at Hutchings. Table 1 shows the domains of functioning that were assessed and the percentages of persons in each age group who reported having difficulties in each domain. Although the older group reported more problems in the physical disabilities category, and both groups reported essentially the same number of problems with personal hygiene, the 18 to 35 group consistently displayed greater difficulty in all other community functioning domains. The younger group had markedly greater problems in the domains of psychiatric symptoms, daily living skills, behavior problems, social isolation, and alcohol and drug abuse problems. It is clear from these data that younger patients are experiencing far more difficulty in navigating community life situations than the older chronic population.

TREATMENT HISTORIES

The treatment careers of the 369 young adult chronic patients identified in 1979 were reviewed at four different points in time over 22 months. At all sample points, nearly 60 per cent of this patient population were receiving some type of inpatient, outpatient, or day treatment service. We also found that a core group of 124, or 34 per cent of the original 369, were enrolled in service on all sample dates. Further review indicated that, in addition to the 34 per cent who were enrolled on all four dates, 49 per cent were intermittently enrolled in service over the 22 months and 17 per cent were not enrolled at all.

We compared a systematic sample of 50 of the persons who were actively enrolled in Hutchings programs during May 1981 with a sample of 55 of those who were not active on any of the four dates. It is important to note that the sample of 50 who were active in May 1981 is a combination of those who were active on all four dates and those who were enrolled intermittently.

No differences between the two groups were revealed with respect to age; in fact, median age differed by only one year for the enrolled and not enrolled groups (26 and 27 years, respectively). The groups were evenly distributed in regard to gender; both groups showed a slight predominance of men—58 per cent for those enrolled and 53 per cent for those not enrolled. When we examined the dimension of ethnicity, however, we detected a significant association between "group" and ethnic status ($\chi^2 = 4.60$, df = 3, $p < .10$). Twenty per cent of the enrolled group were black, while blacks constituted only 7 per cent of those who were not enrolled. Of the other variables examined, we found the most dramatic differences in diagnosis. A significant relationship emerged between enrollment status and the presence or absence of a schizophrenic diagnosis ($\chi^2 = 11.21$, df = 3, $p < .001$). Specifically, only 25 per cent of those not enrolled in any services were diagnosed as schizophrenic while 64 per cent of those actively enrolled were diagnosed as such. This latter percentage is also significantly different from the 25 per cent diagnosed as being schizophrenic in the 18 to 34 age group.

Although we could not secure additional information about the 55 persons who were no longer enrolled, we did obtain additional data about the 50 persons still consuming services at Hutchings. Ninety per cent of these persons were unmarried, more than 75 per cent were unemployed and/or were receiving either public assistance or Supplemental Security Income, and more than 80 per cent were currently using psychotropic drugs. Nearly half of these persons had completed high school and two-thirds lived in their own home or apartment either alone or with family or spouse. This finding is similar to that reported by Lamb and Goertzel (9), which showed that contrary to popular belief, less than one-third of young and chronically disabled individuals in this era of community treatment live in board and care homes or cheap hotels. According to Lamb and Goertzel, most live in nonsegregated, noninstitutionalized settings such as those found in our own study. Finally, more than half of the sample of 50 first entered the Hutchings system when they were between the ages of 13 and 20; 11, or 22 per cent, were found to be developmentally disabled.

The most profound theme emerging from interviews with service providers is that young adults with chronic disabilities may have youth and loneliness in common, but they often differ dramatically from one another.

YOUNG ADULT SUBGROUPS

In a related but independent effort, we sought data which would convey what young adult chronic patients are like as persons and what one would likely experience in a service encounter with them. We interviewed 22 direct service providers from state, county, and voluntary agencies. All of the informants were involved daily with young adult chronic patients.

The most profound theme surfacing from these interviews is that young adults with chronic disabilities may have youth and loneliness in common, but they often differ dramatically from one another. The factors that apparently account for these differences include developmental stage, functional ability, socioeconomic background, and life style.

A content analysis of interviews allowed us to identify both similarities and differences in young chronic patients. From this analysis three distinct groups of patients emerged, each with identifiable characteristics, and each with a full complement of service needs and wants. Table 2 summarizes the characteristics of these groups.

The low-energy, low-demand group. Individuals from this group usually entered a state hospital or state school when they were children or adolescents and thus are already system-dependent. Some may come from backgrounds of social deprivation; others are more fortunate. Nevertheless, they are all well ensconced in the role of patient. Even in remission, they tend to exhibit poor personal hygiene and are generally unkempt. Passivity and low motivation also characterize them. Their environment is circumscribed by the programmatic `watering holes in the mental health system or the social isolation of their homes. Their system dependency is expressed through their concrete attachment to programs and program places. In spite of their youth, these patients appear to be burned out and

TABLE 2 Hypothesized typology of young adult chronic patients

Low-energy, low-demand group	High-energy, high-demand group	High-functioning group
Well ensconced in role of patient	Able to shop around from agency to agency to get what they want	Generally higher socioeconomic status and better appearance
Do not do well, even in remission	Fluctuating functional abilities and interests	New to mental health system
Concretely attached to programs and program places	"Give me what I want or stay out of my life" attitude toward mental health services	Resist mental health program involvement on the basis of conviction
Probably entered mental health system in early adolescence	Low frustration tolerance, acting out, encounters with the law	Some entered mental health system because of alcohol or drug abuse
Passive, poorly motivated	Frequently evicted, mobile	Want to understand their disorders and ways of preventing relapses
Accepting of mental health services	Expectations of self-reliance	Want to blend into general population without being identified as mental patients
Appear burned out at an early age	Includes "revolving door" patients and street people	

to have acquiesced to the directives of mental health service providers in their acceptance of the all-encompassing mental patient status.

The high-energy, high-demand group. Individuals from this group make inordinate demands on case managers. When they want something, either money, discharge papers, or their therapist, they want it right away. And when they don't want psychiatric services, they want their therapists to leave them alone and stay out of their lives. When they feel ignored or neglected, they have the mobility and confrontational skills to shop around from agency to agency until they get what they want. Although they are aggressive on their own behalf, their low frustration tolerance and impulsive behaviors frequently result in encounters with the law. The same impulsivity often culminates in eviction, and when viable housing options have been exhausted, individuals from this group often end up in the streets. Their physical mobility produces financial instability as well. Supplemental Security Income and public assistance checks are often held up or terminated when these patients move without notice from their transient addresses. It is not uncommon for them to lose their public assistance eligibility by taking a job at a fast-food restaurant for two days and then leaving after an explosive encounter with the manager. Members of this group are not without material aspirations; they often spend their limited funds on TVs, stereos, and tape decks. Possessing few sexual inhibitions, they meet one another on inpatient units, fall in love, and bear children. But because of their unstable life styles, their children are most often placed permanently in foster care. This group is characterized by high energy, fluctuating functional abilities, and expectations of self-reliance. However, they are plagued by vacillating moods and interests, which are reflected in their erratic search for services, security, and meaning. Two small but well-known populations within this group are street people and revolving-door patients who generally appear only when destitute or decompensated.

The high-functioning, high-aspiration group.[1] This group is typified by the ability to function at a fairly high level. As a group, they tend to be better educated than the average person in the public mental health system and they most often come from higher income classes. Most are new to the mental health system and frequently arrive because of drug or alcohol abuse. The appearance of these clients contrasts markedly with that of more obviously disabled patients: they are better dressed, apparently healthier, and generally more attractive. However, their appearance can be misleading; these patients are or have been seriously disabled by their disorders and are often without social support. Unlike more dependent institutionalized patients, this group considers planned mental health activities demeaning. They do not want to be identified with traditional mental health programs, older chronic patients, or with peers their own age who are more debilitated than themselves. Their reluctance to engage in traditional mental health programs appears qualitatively different from that of the more erratic group. In contrast to an adolescent rebellion, their resistance seems born of conviction. They are inquisitive and want to exercise control over their lives. They want to know about their condition, about medications and side-effects, and how to prevent relapses. This group clearly expresses neither hopelessness nor helplessness about their disorders; indeed, they feel very keenly their own expectations as well as those of family and staff, and hope to fulfill all of them. What they want

[1] The description of this hypothesized subgroup is derived from an unpublished report on psychosocial rehabilitation programs submitted to the Title 20 training unit of the New York State Office of Mental Health in September 1979 by Sheila LeGacy of Transitional Living Services, Inc., of Syracuse and Edward Benson of Hutchings Psychiatric Center.

most of all is the opportunity to blend into the general population without being identified as mental patients.

The data we have reported are derived from different methodologies and hence are not directly comparable. It is, however, instructive to review their qualitative similarities. A striking congruence exists between the characteristics of the random sample of 50 young adults enrolled in service on all four sample dates and the characteristics of the hypothesized system-dependent group. These patients are consistent, dependent consumers of services and, as the hypothesized narrative and the data suggest, they generally entered the service system as adolescents.

The limited nature of the data prevents us from making specific statements about the congruence between the hypothesized high-functioning group and the sample of patients not enrolled in any Hutchings service. Some speculation, however, is warranted. The hypothesized profile of the high-functioning group indicated that these individuals would perform relatively well during remission. This notion was supported by the less severe diagnoses assigned to those who were not enrolled. In the absence of hard data addressing reasons for the sample groups' lack of participation in Hutchings services, it seems logical that they may well believe traditional mental health services to be demeaning.

Finally, although no empirical data have yet been assembled that verify the existence of the hypothesized high-energy, high-demand group, Schwartz and Goldfinger (10) have published a report supporting the subgroup's existence, and qualitative evidence for the other two subgroups is certainly strong enough to warrant increased attention.

These findings suggest that we should pursue more rigorously the notion of this taxonomy. We may need to alter services and styles of relating to the subgroups in order to provide effective interventions. For example, the system-dependent group may need and accept traditional bench assembly sheltered work; however, the high-functioning group would probably reject it in favor of the more creative vocational programs such as transitional employment placements or employment in a restaurant operating under a vocational evaluation and training certificate. While the most dependent group is likely to accept psychosocial clubs that operate from a single location, the higher functioning group would probably require "clubs without walls"—activities that occur in a variety of community settings including homes, restaurants, and neighborhood pubs. For the erratic group there may be a need for drop-in centers designed for youths, temporary shelters, and day vocational alternatives.

IMPACT ON SERVICES

Although a precise picture of the characteristics and needs of the young adult chronic population is still being formulated, the problems, aspirations, and demands of the group have already challenged our conventional wisdom. In response to this challenge, we will need to think differently about the way we plan and provide treatment, rehabilitation, and community support services.

For example, there is a need to make better use of epidemiological and demographic predictive methods in the planning of mental health systems. We must be able to ascertain how many people in specific age groups with particular problems will need specific types of services. We need to realistically include indefinite-term inpatient and indefinite-term community residence options in the array of comprehensive mental health services. This is to accommodate those patients who do not respond totally to acute-care models of service and who therefore require special health care, protective custody, and security control services.

We must re-educate mental health professionals and paraprofessionals to the principles and practices of chronic care and specifically how it differs from acute-care models of service. It would be essential to convey, for example, that the treatment values of transcendence, independence, normalization, and cure may become myths when inappropriately applied to chronic patients. Precision in understanding and acknowledging the total range of needs of the chronically disabled is also necessary; such precision will enable us to design prescriptive and targeted services. We must learn to accept with hope rather than despair the limits of treatment and the realistic expectations of rehabilitation and indefinite-term community support services. We must design specialized programs that cater to certain age groups, cultures, and disability levels such as drop-in centers for the young and senior citizen club programs for the aged. There is also a need to adapt our clinical styles of relating to this population and to become more willing to enter life enterprises with these patients. And finally, assuming we are entering a new era and will make mistakes along the way, we need to establish our programs in a manner that implicitly includes evaluation of them.

CONCLUSIONS

In our varied work settings there is an opportunity to embrace the challenge of young adult chronic patients and to expand our imaginations in designing systems to serve them. Before we begin, however, there are two themes suggested by data presented here.

First, as we design programs for young adult chronic patients, let us do so with a clear idea of how these patients are alike as individuals and as a group and how they are different. Second, let us seize the opportunity to set up our programs in such a way that every program change and every service innovation may be evaluated. Only by developing this data-based information will we be able to look back and accurately assess the impact of our services on the disorder, the duration of stay, the life functioning, and the life satisfaction of this group.■

REFERENCES

1) Pepper B, Kirshner M, Ryglewicz H: The young adult chronic patient: overview of a population. Hospital & Community Psychiatry 32:463–469, 1981

2) Shore MF, Shapiro R: The effects of deinstitutionalization on the state hospital. Hospital & Community Psychiatry 30:605–608, 1979

3) Cotton PG, Bene-Kociemba A, Cole R: The effect of deinstitutionalization on a general hospital's psychiatric unit. Hospital & Community Psychiatry 30:609–612, 1979

4) Kramer M: Population changes and schizophrenia: 1970–1985. Presented at the second Rochester International Conference on Schizophrenia, held in Rochester, NY, May 1976

5) Pepper B, Ryglewicz H: The young adult chronic patient, keynote address: overview of the population and the issues. Presented at the Conference on the Young Adult Chronic Patient held in Suffern, NY, Nov 20–21, 1980

6) Minkoff K: A map of chronic patients, in The Chronic Mental Patient. Edited by Talbott JA. Washington, DC, American Psychiatric Association, 1978

7) Goldman HH, Gattozzi AA, Taube CA: Defining and counting the chronically mentally ill. Hospital & Community Psychiatry 32:21–27, 1981

8) Wing JK: Who becomes chronic. Psychiatric Quarterly 50:178–190, 1978

9) Lamb RH, Goertzel V: The long-term patient in the era of community treatment. Archives of General Psychiatry 34:679–682, 1977

10) Schwartz S, Goldfinger S: The new chronic patient: clinical characteristics of an emerging subgroup. Hospital & Community Psychiatry 32:470–474, 1981

Young Adult Chronic Patients: The New Drifters

H. RICHARD LAMB, M.D.
Professor of Psychiatry
University of Southern California School of Medicine
Los Angeles, California

Young chronic patients are faced with the same concerns and life-cycle stresses as others in their age group. They strive for independence, satisfying relationships, a sense of identity, and a realistic vocational choice. Lacking the ability to withstand stress and intimacy, they struggle and often repeatedly fail. The result is anxiety, depression, psychotic episodes, and hospitalizations; gradually many begin to give up the struggle. Such concerns may become intensified during the reassessment of life that takes place at about age 30. Denial of illness, the rebelliousness of youth, and issues of control and violence compound the problems. Since deinstitutionalization, patients can no longer take asylum from stresses in a lifetime of hospitalization. Many patients drift from one city to another, or from one living situation to another. Some ways of approaching these problems, such as working with younger patients while they may still be motivated to make changes, helping them develop appropriate rationalizations, and supporting realistic goals, are discussed.

■In the universal search for meaning in life, many long-term severely disabled psychiatric patients find only emptiness. A positive sense of meaning in life is usually associated with membership in groups, dedication to some cause, and adoption of clear life goals (1). In all these areas, long-term patients generally fall short.

A recent study of long-term severely disabled psychiatric patients (in a board-and-care home in Los Angeles) showed that significantly more patients under age 30 than over age 30 had goals to change something in their lives (2). What does this finding mean? Perhaps, as these persons with limited capabilities become older, they have experienced repeated failures in dealing with life's demands and in achieving their earlier goals. They have had more time to lower or set aside their goals, and to accept a life without goals and a low level of functioning that does not exceed their capabilities. In the same study, a strong relationship was found between age and history of hospitalization; three-fourths of those under age 30 had been hospitalized during the preceding year, compared with only one-fifth over age 30.

Dr. Lamb's address is USC Department of Psychiatry, 1934 Hospital Place, Los Angeles, California 90033.

Young people who are just beginning to deal with life's demands and to make their way in the world are struggling to achieve a measure of independence, to choose and succeed at a vocation, to establish satisfying interpersonal relationships and attain some degree of intimacy, and to acquire some sense of identity. Because the mentally ill person lacks ego strength, the ability to withstand stress, and the ability to form meaningful interpersonal relationships, his efforts often lead only to failure. The result may be a still more determined, even frantic, effort with a greatly increased level of anxiety that begins to border on desperation. Ultimately, such anxiety may lead to another failure, accompanied by feelings of despair. For a person predisposed to retreat into psychosis, repeated failures lead to a stormy course with acute psychotic breaks and hospitalizations. The situation becomes compounded when such persons are in an environment where unrealistic expectations emanate not just from within themselves, but also from families and mental health professionals.

Some chronically dysfunctional and mentally disordered individuals gradually, over a period of years, succeed in their strivings for independence, a vocation, intimacy, and a sense of identity. Many others, however, eventually give up the struggle and find face-saving rationalizations for their limited degree of functioning and accomplishments. For instance, a middle-aged woman says, "I would have raised my children, but the judge was lied to and took them away from me." Or someone in his middle years says, "I am retired now on Social Security," when in fact he receives Supplemental Security Income because of his disabling psychiatric disorder. Similar rationalizations come from chronically dysfunctional persons who have come to feel they must passively submit to overwhelming forces that control their destinies and impede their progress. Often one eventually hears no rationalizations at all but finds only a constricted passive stance on life. An example would be the patient who seems to look no further than his next cigarette.

Thus, as patients age, much of the pressure that had resulted in psychotic decompensations is removed. Maturation also seems a factor, since age makes people less impulsive and "more philosophical" in the face of adversity and disappointment.

FACING THE CRISIS OF AGE 30

Chronically disabled patients in both the younger and older age groups are disheartened and depressed, just as we all would be, about not having goals, about not being able to reach goals, about experiencing repeated failures instead. Concerns about getting older with little to show for one's life are felt not only by those in the involutional period but also by those who are approaching age 30 and even by those still in their mid-twenties.

As one approaches and then reaches 30, there is inevitably a process of assessing one's achievements, or lack of them, and of the extent to which goals set for this age have been reached. Nearing age 30 seems to be a time of settling down, a time for taking life more seriously and giving up the "frivolities" of youth, a time to marry or to establish a permanent relationship, to be at least launched on a career, and to consolidate one's plans. When the assessment of one's life at this age is not positive, many feel that life has not been worthwhile, and are beset by feelings of inadequacy and depression. This point may seem self-evident, and yet all too often there is a tendency to forget that long-term, severely mentally ill patients are affected by the stresses and concerns of each phase of the life cycle, and that they have the same existential concerns as do we all.

Before deinstitutionalization these patients, who have been called the new chronic patients, were chronically institutionalized, often at the time of their first break in adolescence or early adulthood. Sometimes they improved in the hospital and were discharged, but at their next decompensation were rehospitalized, never to return to the community. Thus after their initial failures in trying to cope with the vicissitudes of life and of living in the community, they were no longer exposed to these stresses: they were given permanent asylum from the demands of the world.

Now hospital stays tend to be brief. In this sense, the majority of the new long-term patients are the products of deinstitutionalization. This is not to imply that we should turn the clock back and return to a system of total institutionalization for all long-term patients. In the community these patients can have something very precious—their liberty, to the extent they can handle it. Further, if we provide the resources, they can realize their potential for successfully passing some of life's milestones.

Only three decades ago there were no psychotropic drugs to bring such persons out of their world of autistic fantasy and put reality into clearer perspective. It was also more difficult to return them to the community. Even today many patients fail to take their psychotropic medications in order to avoid the dysphoric feelings of depression and anxiety that result when they see their reality too clearly; they prefer grandiosity and a blurring of reality to a relative drug-induced normality (3). Psychoactive drugs help prevent long-term hospitalization, which previously kept long-term patients from trying to find a place for themselves in the world. But, similarly, drugs have denied to many the simple, more immediate gratification of long-term asylum from stress.

A large proportion of new chronic patients tend to deny a need for mental health treatment (4). Admitting mental illness seems to them to be admitting failure. Many feel that becoming part of the mental health system is like joining an army of misfits (5). Instead, many medicate themselves with street drugs; thus they also gain admittance to the drug subculture, where they can find acceptance despite their lack of status in the conventional sense.

Another factor contributing to these patients' refusal of treatment is the natural rebelliousness of youth, a normal part of the process of striving for independence and autonomy; one feels a sense of independence when taking a position at the other extreme from parents or society generally (or, in this instance, from the mental health establishment). In the normal course of events, someone who feels more secure in his independence can begin to moderate his positions without feeling that he has lost his new-found independence. With most long-term patients, it is a lack of readiness for independence, which the patient may or may not be able to acknowledge, and of which he may not even be aware, that sooner or later necessitates his accepting patienthood.

If we do not keep these dynamics in mind, and even if we do, we may find the young chronic patients provocative and aggravating (6). A usual response of mental health professionals is to find a way to prematurely terminate their treatment.

ISSUES OF CONTROL AND VIOLENCE

An important problem in working with younger psychotic patients is dealing with issues of control and violence. In a study of persons sent to a state hospital over a four-month period from a California county that attempts to treat as many patients as possible in local inpatient facilities, it was found that 60 per cent of the patients had a recent history of physical violence in the community or in the local facility that transferred them to the state hospital (7). When only males (median age, 24.5 years) in the study were considered, the figure rose to 71 per cent. In another study, in a locked facility in which the median age was 25, a total of 41 per cent of the patients had been physically assaultive to other persons within the preceding 12 months (8).

Thus, for a relatively small but important group of younger patients, there are difficult problems of control and management in community settings. Many of these patients are characterized by assaultive behavior, severe overt psychopathology, lack of internal controls, reluctance to take psychotropic medications, an inability to adjust to open settings, problems with drugs and

Young chronic patients become drifters for many reasons: to leave problems and failures behind, to try to find, or avoid, closeness, to search for autonomy, or to avoid involvement in a treatment program.

alcohol in addition to their psychoses, and, in some cases, self-destructive behavior. They often require highly structured community settings such as locked skilled nursing facilities or extended stays in state hospitals.

Assessing the need for external control and structure is extremely important. When an attempt is made to manage such patients in less structured community settings, as in community mental health programs, these patients, though relatively few in numbers, tend to take up an inordinate share of the time and effort of mental health professionals. Further, although acting out defiantly, rebelliously, and violently may be an attempt to achieve independence and individuation, the community may not be able to tolerate the actions of these patients who do not demonstrate sufficient self-control.

Often overlooked by professionals are the effects of the violent acts on the patients who have committed them, especially if the victim is a close relative, friend, or caretaker. The aftermath may be a web of guilt and remorse that only compounds the patient's problems. Further, the realization of having already lost control and the fear that it may happen again can be extremely anxiety-provoking.

THE NEW DRIFTERS

"Drifter" is a word that strikes a chord in all those who have contact with young, chronic patients—mental health professionals, families, and the patients themselves. Some drifters wander from community to community seeking a geographic solution to their problems; hoping to leave their problems behind, they find that they have simply brought their difficulties to a new location. Others drift in the community from one living situation to another, and some, though they remain in one place, can best be described as drifting through life: they lead a life without goals, direction, or ties other than perhaps a hostile-dependent relationship with parents or other caretakers.

Why do they drift? In addition to their desire to outrun their problems, their symptoms, and their failures, they have great difficulty achieving closeness and intimacy. A fantasy of finding closeness elsewhere encourages them to move on. Yet all too often if they stumble into an intimate relationship or find themselves in a residence where there is caring and closeness and sharing, the increased anxiety they experience creates a need to run.

They drift also in search of autonomy, as a way of denying their dependency and out of a desire for an isolated life style. And they drift because of a reluctance to become involved in a mental health treatment program or a supportive out-of-home environment, such as a halfway house or board-and-care home, that would give them a mental patient identity and make them part of the mental health system; they do not want to see themselves as ill.

Let us consider, for example, those who move from one community residence to another. Many of them may be trying to escape the pull of dependency and may not be ready to come to terms with living in a sheltered, segregated, low-pressure environment. Those who move on are more apt to still have life goals (9); some may see leaving their comparatively static milieu as a necessary part of the process of realizing their goals.

The group who tend not to move about—for instance, who stay on in a board-and-care home—are older and are less likely to have goals for themselves; fewer have been hospitalized during the preceding year (9). In general, it would appear that this group has settled into the routine of board-and-care life, given up whatever earlier goals they may have had, and settled for a more limited existence. Using incidence of hospitalization as the criterion, they have stabilized to a greater degree. They seem to have given in to the pull of dependency, having weighed the costs of striving for independence and achievement against giving up, which poses less risk of failure, stress, and decompensation.

APPROACHING THE PROBLEMS

What can be done to begin to resolve the problems of the new, young, long-term patient? Obviously establishing an array of high-quality community treatment and rehabilitation resources is a crucial first step. We now know enough about the kinds of resources that are most effective for these patients, and mental health decision-makers are beginning to see that these patients should receive our highest priority. But in the meantime, we must not be carried away by goals of mainstreaming and normalization when such goals are unrealistic, and must recognize that we can contribute a great deal to the lives of long-term patients whether or not they are capable of becoming fully functioning members of our society, socially and vocationally. Improving the quality of life for these patients is an important objective, in and of itself.

What about the young chronic patients for whom life seems to hold no meaning? Engagement is the therapeutic answer to meaninglessness (1). To quote Yalom: "To find a home, to care about other individuals, about ideas or projects, to search, to create, to build—these, and all other forms of engagement, are twice rewarding: they are intrinsically enriching, and they alleviate the dysphoria that stems from being bombarded with the unassembled brute data in existence." Engagement is the answer, too, for the new drifters, though the extent to which they can become engaged will vary greatly.

It is especially important to work intensively with younger patients while they still have goals, have had less time to settle into a life of regression, and, one hopes, are still motivated to make changes in their lives. We must be sure that their goals, and ours, are realistic. For instance, if the limits of a patient's capabilities are a sheltered workshop or at best an entry-level job, we should support this endeavor. Such an activity might seem demeaning to us, or might seem inappropriate to us for an intelligent patient from an achieving family, but it might well give the patient a feeling of productivity and self-respect he has never known before. We must be sure that the pace is one the patient can handle, and must not let his impatience, or ours, propel him onto a fast track to failure. And we must provide, or help him find, sufficient supports during this difficult period.

We have discussed these young persons' quest for autonomy, their fear of being labeled as psychiatric misfits, and the reluctance of many to accept our services. In many cases we can persuade them to enter our programs. But in many others we cannot (10). Unless someone's behavior becomes so self-destructive that his safety and well-being are compromised, or his behavior becomes more destructive or disruptive than society can tolerate, we must often learn to wait until maturity has shifted the balance, or he has found some way to rationalize his turning to us. If we have an opportunity to see patients over long periods of time, we may find that we must wait for years, through repeated crises and many attempts to involve the patient with us.

It is important that we try to minimize our disappointment if our offers of help are rejected; we need to accept that our powers of persuasion are limited. Otherwise our feelings of disappointment are communicated to the patient, who experiences them as a sign that he has failed to measure up again. We also need to focus on the problems and concerns of becoming 30. Thus we should offer programs, within the patient's capabilities, to help him acquire a vocational identity. We should respond to the patient's assessment of himself as a person who cannot cope by offering supports such as living arrangements geared to his needs, psychotropic drugs, and a stable source of income. In these ways we can help to stabilize the patient's life in the community and demonstrate to him that it is within *his* power, by accepting these supports, to eliminate the chaos in his life. At the same time it is important for the patient to see that everyone, not just psychiatric patients, needs a support system to cope with life's demands.

Helping the patient develop rationalizations will sometimes facilitate his adjustment. For instance, one can help him delay entry into situations beyond his capabilities, such as a demanding vocational program or a more independent living situation, by encouraging him to see the delay as part of his convalescence from a "nervous breakdown," or from a period of years "out in the cold." Such a delay may or may not be temporary. But even if it turns out to be permanent, it has been a face-saving way for the patient to avoid a situation he could not handle. He has been spared a psychotic episode or the need to run, or drift, away from his treatment. Later the problem can be dealt with in a more definitive way.

Who among us faces all of the realities of our lives without the use of rationalization? If one examines the therapy of healthier patients, one finds it is usually considered successful if the patient comes to terms with the realities of his life. And that usually means he rationalizes to some degree, not simply that he faces squarely all the stark realities of his past, his present, and his future.

Finally, the importance of the one-to-one relationship between trained helping professionals and their patients should not be forgotten. This is an age in which the treatment of long-term patients often consists of psychotropic drugs accompanied only by "coordination" by relatively untrained persons of services that may or may not exist, or may or may not be possible to coordinate. We should keep in mind the capabilities, or lack of them, of our patients, and their reactions to the stresses of the life cycle and their failures to meet their own and society's expectations. And we should provide professionals trained to listen, trained to assess patients' capabilities, trained to reinforce patients' rationalizations when it is appropriate, trained to encourage productivity when it is possible, and trained to help patients find their own level of independence, engagement, and personal dignity.■

REFERENCES

1) Yalom ID: Existential Psychotherapy. New York, Basic Books, 1980

2) Lamb HR: The new asylums in the community. Archives of General Psychiatry 36:129–134, 1979

3) Van Putten T, Crumpton E, Yale C: Drug refusal in schizophrenia and the wish to be crazy. Archives of General Psychiatry 33:1443–1446, 1976

4) Pepper B, Kirshner MC, Ryglewicz H: The young adult chronic patient: overview of a population. Hospital & Community Psychiatry 32:463–469, 1981

5) Estroff SE: Making It Crazy: An Ethnography of Psychiatric Clients in an American Community. Los Angeles, University of California Press, 1981, pp 250–253

6) Schwartz SR, Goldfinger SM: The new chronic patient: clinical characteristics of an emerging subgroup. Hospital & Community Psychiatry 32:470–474, 1981

7) Lamb HR: The state hospital: facility of last resort. American Journal of Psychiatry 134:1151–1152, 1977

8) Lamb HR: Structure: the neglected ingredient of community treatment. Archives of General Psychiatry 37:1224–1228, 1980

9) Lamb HR: Board-and-care home wanderers. Archives of General Psychiatry 37:135–137, 1980

10) Bachrach LL: Young adult chronic patients: an analytical review of the literature. Hospital & Community Psychiatry 33:189–197, 1982

The Young Adult Chronic Patient: Overview of a Population

BERT PEPPER, M.D.
Director
MICHAEL C. KIRSHNER, PH.D.
Director of Professional Education and Training
HILARY RYGLEWICZ, A.C.S.W.
Clinical Assistant to the Director
Rockland County Community Mental Health Center
Pomona, New York

A new generation of persistently dysfunctional young adults (aged 18 to 35) has emerged in the community, requiring new programs in community care. This population, which includes a wide range of diagnostic groups, is under study at a suburban New York community mental health center. The center and county are serving 294 such young patients through a variety of programs which include a crisis service, a sheltered workshop, a residential program called the Community Link-Up Experience, an acute day treatment program, an alcohol day treatment program, a case management program, and a Growth Advancement Program that gives patients an opportunity to socialize and share problems with others their age. Residential programs that provide a supportive living situation to young adult chronic patients on both a temporary and a long-term basis are sorely needed and will require an increased outlay of funds. A case study of one young patient who visited the center sporadically over a 12-year period illustrates the treatment problems such patients pose.

■Much has been said and written about the direct effect of deinstitutionalization in the United States. The reduction of the population of state and county mental hospitals nationwide from 558,922 in 1955 to 159,405 in 1977 (1) is evidenced by the emergence of shopping-bag ladies, by the growth of the single-room-occupancy hotel, proprietary (board-and-care) home, and nursing home industries, and by the overload on community mental health and state aftercare programs.

The purpose of this article is to raise the consciousness of mental health professionals to the other side of deinstitutionalization: the emergence of a population of young adult chronic patients who have spent relatively little time in hospitals but who present persistent and frustrating problems to community caregivers in mental health and other social service systems. We are referring to people between the ages of 18 and 30 or 35 who are psychiatrically and socially impaired, so seriously that they are continually or recurrently clients of mental health and other social service agencies over a period of years.

Diagnostically, these young adults carry a variety of labels—schizophrenia, other psychoses, and personality disorders prominent among them. Although they present a variety of symptom profiles, they share two overarching characteristics: their severe difficulties in social functioning, and their tendency to use mental health services inappropriately, in ways that drain the time and energy of clinicians yet do not conform to viable treatment plans.

Two decades ago Ernest Gruenberg began publishing a brilliant series of reports of patients in our state hospitals who, despite a variety of diagnoses, could commonly be described as suffering from a "social breakdown syndrome" (2–9). Their behavior was characterized by poor social and psychological functioning, apathy, negativism, and docility mingled with episodic outbursts—seemingly the contribution of institutional life to their behavior, as also chronicled by Goffman (10). However a decade ago Gruenberg observed the syndrome in individuals who had not had long residence in an institution.

Many in our patient group are less frequently and consistently disabled than Gruenberg's patients, and a high proportion have never required hospitalization. But social breakdown syndrome is one of the dysfunctional patterns we have observed in this, our first generation of chronically impaired, young adult patients who have spent little or no time in mental hospitals.

When such young adults appear in our emergency rooms, hospital admission is a last resort. Our involuntary admissions must meet stricter legal standards than in the past; our voluntary admissions must withstand more careful scrutiny. Diversion of such patients to a day program or other outpatient treatment is a likely suggestion, but one that is often not accepted or not

Dr. Pepper is also clinical professor of psychiatry at New York University School of Medicine in New York City. The authors' address is Rockland County Community Mental Health Center, Pomona, New York 10970. This overview is based on papers presented by the authors at a conference on "The Young Adult Chronic Patient: Clinical and Programmatic Issues" sponsored by the Rockland County Community Mental Health Center November 20–21, 1980, in Suffern, New York. It is the first in a series of four papers on the new chronic patient published in this issue.

followed by these help-seeking yet help-rejecting young people. If they are admitted to the hospital, their stays are measured in days or weeks rather than months, years, or decades.

Young adult chronic patients living in the community are socially and psychologically different from older deinstitutionalized patients, and from those never-institutionalized, older adult chronic patients who are sometimes included among "new chronics." Younger patients are different because failure is new to them; because they are still struggling to be like their age-mates; because they have not learned, as have deinstitutionalized patients, to be docile and do as they are told; because they act out—many take drugs—in the manner of withdrawn or rebellious youth; and because they are as likely to blame mental health professionals as they are to turn to them for help.

The functional criteria we have used in defining this group cut across diagnostic and programmatic lines. We are conducting an informal exploratory study at the Rockland County Community Mental Health Center with input from more than 100 clinicians on our interdisciplinary staff. Approximately 900 patients in the age group 18 to 30 were identified as having been served in the three-month period from June through August 1980. Of these 900, a total of 294 were categorized by clinicians and through chart review as members of the group we have called young adult chronic patients. They were readily identifiable as having a characteristic configuration of functional disabilities and of treatment and social service needs. Slightly more than half, 165, are males.

On our records, these 294 patients carry 40 different specific diagnoses. Nearly two-thirds, or 192 patients, have a diagnosis of major mental illness. Of the 294 patients, 169 were diagnosed as schizophrenic, with 97 diagnosed as having schizophrenia, chronic undifferentiated type. Twenty-one others had a primary diagnosis of major affective disorder (manic-depressive illness), while two others had an atypical or other psychosis. The remainder had the primary diagnoses of personality disorders (36 patients), behavior disorders (16 patients), neuroses (24 patients), drug dependence or alcohol abuse (10 patients), and organic brain syndrome, mental retardation, or specific learning disability (16 patients).

CLINICAL IMPRESSIONS

The variety of diagnoses in our group indicates the need to view these young chronic patients functionally rather than in terms of their labels. The treatment needs implied by the specific diagnoses must be met, of course. But the presenting disturbances of these young adults and their social and treatment needs are disconcertingly similar, for they spring from the problems all these patients have in common: their acute vulnerability to stress, their difficulty in making stable and supportive relationships, their inability to get and keep something good in their lives, and their repeated failures of judgment, which can be seen as an inability or refusal to learn from their experiences.

These patients provoke an uncommon amount of frustration and distress, not only from their relatives and associates but also from their clinicians and caseworkers. They confound our efforts to treat them by conventional means, they evade yet repeatedly disturb our mental health programs, and they appear again and again in our psychiatric emergency services and police stations. Some, though not all, sojourn briefly in our psychiatric hospitals, where their names are likely to be well known, where they consume disproportionate quantities of staff time, where, like recalcitrant children, they create more than their share of consternation, where they are the subject of multiple case presentations and interagency treatment planning conferences—only to be discharged back into lives that often prove once again untenable.

These patients rarely reward our efforts with improvement. Instead they become, individually and collectively, our albatross. They are functioning persons only in a marginal sense; they manage their lives tenuously at best and disastrously at worst. They are discharged when their most acute symptoms have abated, but typically their remissions are incomplete.

PRELIMINARY DATA

A majority (68 per cent of our 294 patients) are still living with parents or "others," which often means other patients met in hospitals or drug programs. A minority (17 per cent) live alone, which often means they are perpetual transients through the cheerless halls of single-room-occupancy hotels. The remaining 15 per cent live in community residences (9 per cent), proprietary homes (3 per cent), or family care (3 per cent). A majority (57 per cent) depend on some form of public assistance, and many (19 per cent) are still supported by their parents; only 24 per cent are self-supporting.

Most have been able to make only transient, unstable, unsatisfactory relationships with people their own age; their friends and lovers are often other marginally functional people with equally uneven life courses and dubious prognoses. A sizable number abuse alcohol (37 per cent) or other drugs (37 per cent—not necessarily the same 37 per cent); some of them are quite obviously self-medicating to dull the pain of their confusion and despair. At least 24 per cent have been in trouble with the law, usually in ways clearly related to their emotional and social impairment. A high proportion (42 per cent) present a risk of suicide, for reasons that certainly include the simple fact that they see no hope for the future.

A DEVELOPMENTAL PERSPECTIVE

The words "young" and "chronic" joined together make an unpleasant phrase. Indeed, the word "chronic" is misleading and prejudicial, for a minority of these patients are eventually able to pursue fairly normal lives, and for many more the term "chronicity" may reflect merely the undeveloped state of our own arts. But these patients are, in a sense, chronically young. They are stuck in the transition from childhood dependence to adult independence, from parental or quasi-parental support to self-supporting work, adult autonomy, and an expanding network of relationships—the fundamental amenities that keep our own lives going.

Like the parents of mentally retarded young people, the parents of young chronic patients wonder, "Who will look after him when I die?" Some of the patients simply remain, figuratively and sometimes literally, home in bed. Some are wanderers. Some become known as troublemakers. Some of them try, again and again, with diminishing hopes, to take some step toward greater independence, or at least more stable functioning. Again and again they fall back into the reluctant yet retentive embrace of their parents, back to the arms of psychiatric and social service systems. Too often they slip through our willing but clumsy fingers, until some new calamity brings them once again to our attention.

A 'HOMELESS' GENERATION

Just as Gruenberg looked at the contribution of institutional life to social breakdown syndrome, we must explore the roles played by the family and society in the formation and persistence of our young chronic patients' repetitive behavior. For those whose behavior springs from the ego deficits involved in serious mental or emotional illness, we also have to reflect that this is the first generation of mental patients to have to cope, from the beginning and during most of their lives, with the tasks and the stresses of community living.

The career of mental patient used to offer, like army life and like some families, at least a measure of stability to make up for the disadvantage of confinement. Our mental hospitals were built and peopled on the assumption that mental patients needed protection from society, just as society needed protection from them. Lately the life course of patients has become much more fluctuating and uncertain.

Of our group of 294, at least 55 per cent received mental health treatment before the age of 18. These were emotionally troubled youngsters who grew up to be chronically dependent young adults. They may have functioned fairly well in childhood and even part way through adolescence, only to become symptomatic when confronting the task of separating from families and achieving an adult identity. They have no refuge to enter now, as deinstitutionalization has rendered many of them essentially homeless.

We estimate that, for every dysfunctional young adult we see, there are two to ten in the community who never arrive at our doorstep but are hidden in dysfunctional families or in jails, or wander unnoticed in our city streets. In a recent conference on the young adult chronic patient sponsored by our center, data on a New York City population of young chronic patients showed an appalling rate of death by suicide—five in one year from a group of 119 patients newly discharged from a state hospital (11). In a moderate-size and richly served community like Rockland County, young chronic patients tend to be more visible and somewhat less at risk.

SELF-PERCEPTIONS

These young adults more often describe themselves to us as social casualties than as victims of mental illness or personality disorders, just as they prefer to remember an episode of disorganized thinking as the result of an incidental ingestion of drugs—the fabled "bad trip"—rather than as an upsurge of psychosis. Many do not define themselves as mental patients, and this, of course, is one of the intended benefits of their being in the community.

But this benefit has other implications. Impaired young adults who do not view themselves as patients are reluctant to acknowledge an ongoing need for medication, and are resistant to seeing themselves as particularly vulnerable to the alcohol, marijuana, and other mind-altering drugs enjoyed recreationally by their age-mates. They sense, quite correctly, that weekly one-to-one therapy is insufficient or irrelevant to their needs; those who do establish a relationship with a therapist may fail to keep appointments when feeling well, yet present themselves on impulse, demanding and indeed requiring attention on a crisis basis. On the other hand, they frequently reject day programs, saying "That's not for me," "I'm going to get a job and make some money," "I'm going to go back to school," or "Those people are all too sick for me. I'm not that sick!"

This reluctance to see themselves as different from anyone else functions as a barrier to accepting treatment. Yet their persistent lack of success in achieving the goals that are socially appropriate to their age—education, mating, a steady job—does set them apart in their own despairing perception, not as patients or impaired people with special needs, but as social failures. Viewing themselves as "just like anybody else," they have to experience, again and again, the pain of difference, the despair of failure. They take refuge from this perception by acting out, by aggressive outbursts, by taking drugs, by taking to their beds, and by blaming and raging against their parents, their landlords, their therapists, the police, the hospital, and society.

A CASE STUDY

An example of the patient group we are describing is a young man we will call Mr. J, who has been known to our center for 12 years. He first came to one of our outpatient clinics in 1968 at age 18, complaining of "failure to meet with school requirements, due to my feelings about people I deal with. . . . School puts me uptight." At that time he was still in high school, where he had been doing poorly since early adolescence. He was living at home with his mother, whom he described as "overworried about everything, always complaining and pressuring me." His father, "a cold and violent person," had been out of the home for two years. The patient was described in the psychiatric evaluation as showing a classic disturbance in thinking, affect, and relating to others and a very disturbed communication system. There was also tentative evidence of paranoid symptomatology.

Mr. J was diagnosed as schizophrenic, chronic undifferentiated type. Since his only effective communication seemed to be with his peers, adolescent group therapy was recommended, to be started after a period of preparation. The next entry in Mr. J's chart is a copy of a letter from his therapist: "Dear Mr. J: I'm sorry you have been unable to keep your appointments with me. . . ." In response to the letter, the patient's mother appeared at the center, worried and tearful, saying that her son was her whole life, but that "he just sleeps all day and doesn't go to school or work." After numerous attempts to engage Mr. J in treatment, his case was closed until he initiated further contact.

The next 11 years of Mr. J's history as a patient in our system include the following events:

In 1971 he requested admission to our inpatient unit, where a friend was hospitalized and where Mr. J felt he could "talk to someone." He complained of having no place to go. He was using heroin, speed, and marijuana and was seen by our staff as anxious and withdrawn but not in need of hospitalization. He was referred back to the outpatient clinic, which he attended during the next several months, breaking many appointments and showing up at unscheduled times. He became belligerent and actively paranoid, and thioridazine was prescribed. He contracted hepatitis caused by his use of heroin. In April 1971 his case was closed again because he refused help of any kind.

In 1972 Mr. J was arrested for armed robbery, which was probably related to his use of drugs. Six months later he appeared at the clinic, stating he had had methadone treatment but now felt jumpy and craved heroin. He was taking 10 mg of diazepam t.i.d., prescribed by his family doctor, and was also drinking. He complained of being unable to build a relationship with a girl. Following this visit he kept no further appointments, despite many efforts to contact him.

In 1974 Mr. J again requested admission as an inpatient, saying he couldn't stand living at home. He was offered admission to the day hospital. He promised to return later to begin the program, but did not return for two years.

For a six-month period in 1976, Mr. J became a habitual user and abuser of the center's emergency service, calling the service frequently to complain of physical symptoms, depression, and boredom. He was referred to the county's social rehabilitation service (now the community support center, described below) and attended for only one day, continuing to call the emergency service. He was clearly decompensating and was addicted to diazepam. Once he called to say he had taken pills and wine and had broken up a girl's apartment "for revenge." A week later a bomb threat to the mental health center was made in a voice that sounded like Mr. J's although he hotly denied making the call.

Mr. J became a habitual user and abuser of the center's emergency service, calling the service frequently to complain of physical symptoms, depression, and boredom.

In 1977 and 1978 the patient formed a relationship with a therapist at the clinic and also began attending the acute day treatment program. He was still taking 5 to 20 mg of diazepam daily, prescribed by several general practitioners. He continued to take the drug after a brief, voluntary admission to our inpatient unit for detoxification.

By 1979 Mr. J had left day treatment and was willing only to continue with his outpatient therapist, but even there his contacts were increasingly sporadic. He was referred to a new center program for young adults (the Growth Advancement Program, described below) but did not attend. He attended some Alcoholics Anonymous meetings, but continued to use diazepam. When a more structured program was again suggested, he became angry with his therapist and walked out.

In 1980 he was hospitalized involuntarily in our inpatient unit following a call from someone in the community who reported that he was expressing paranoid, suicidal, and homicidal ideation. He showed classic symptoms of thought disorder and was preoccupied with relationships that seemed largely based on fantasy. He had recently had his 30th birthday, and learning that a friend a few years older had died, he suspected suicide. He saw himself as following a similar life course.

Unfortunately, this story has neither climax nor ending. At discharge clinicians again urged Mr. J to attend a residential program and to resume day treatment and vocational training. He refused all these options, and although he said he wanted his life to be different, he was unable to undertake change. He continues to live with his mother, to be unemployed and socially isolated, and to abuse drugs in order to assuage the anxiety and tension he lives with constantly. At 30 he has the despairing sense that his life will never change.

HOW ARE WE RESPONDING?

We wanted to find out where young adult chronic patients in Rockland County are now being treated and how we can serve them more effectively. We have the advantages, both in research and in treatment, of an extensive, multiprogram system of service. The Rockland County Community Mental Health Center, which began as a federally constructed and funded facility, comprises more than 50 separate programs. In recent years it has become the core agency of a unified service network for the total care and treatment of the mentally ill, mentally retarded, developmentally disabled, and alcoholic and drug-abusing residents in our county of 270,000 persons.

We have had mixed success in ensuring that our young chronic patients actually use the services available to them. The crisis service is a typical point of entry. Besides a full range of immediate and intensive crisis interventions at the center or in the home, it offers short-term treatment in frequent sessions over several weeks. This brief intensive treatment functions as one alternative to hospitalization for a disturbed young adult. Twenty-three of our patients have recently been treated by the crisis service although they are not involved in other programs—usually because they reject outpatient treatment and do not meet legal standards for hospitalization.

The inpatient unit is a short-term, crisis-oriented unit (mean stay, 17 days) that focuses on rapid resolution of severe presenting programs and return to the community. Often in the course of a hospitalization, a young adult who has remained dependent on his family is encouraged to move toward greater independence, and in some cases to move out of the family home by applying for public assistance and seeking new living quarters while still in the hospital. Our records show that 41 of our group of 294 have been hospitalized one or more times in our inpatient unit but are not currently involved in any of our outpatient programs. Another 178 patients have had one or more hospitalizations (on our inpatient unit or elsewhere) but are recorded as having been seen most recently in an outpatient program.

A minority of our young adult population are referred to the Community Link-Up Experience (CLUE), a 20-bed, two-phase residential program operated by the Rockland Hospital Guild, on the grounds of Rockland Psychiatric Center. The program offers housing to both young adults and older patients who are involved in a day program or other all-day activity. During the first phase patients live in CLUE's halfway house, and in the second phase they share private apartments also located on the grounds. The CLUE program is an example of the kind of supportive residential placement that we believe is sorely needed. Many young chronic patients could benefit from such alternative living arrangements because they simply do not function alone in the community or make, without intensive support, the kind of steady relationships that enable them to work out arrangements with roommates.

Our acute day treatment (day hospital) program is used as a transition from a short-term hospitalization or as an alternative to admission (12). It offers a structured 14-week experience, four days a week, and includes daily group therapy and educational and recreational activities, as well as individual and family therapy and chemotherapy when indicated. Thirty-eight of the 300 patients are presently being served by this program.

Staff consider acute day treatment and its counterpart, the alcohol day treatment program, the treatment of choice for many young adult chronic patients. But, as might be expected, many whom we try to refer will not accept such intensive, all-day programs.

The services of our outpatient clinic range from weekly individual or group therapy to medication visits and also include crisis and walk-in services. The six branch clinics have the advantage of being conveniently located in various neighborhoods in the county. Currently 145 patients are being seen in the clinics. But the services were not designed for our young adult chronic patients, and are often inadequate or inappropriate to their needs. Yet the link to an outpatient clinic is often the single support that young patients will accept.

Many young patients use the services of the outpatient clinic only sporadically or temporarily. Others may try to use the clinic for years of support, draining the time and energy of a single clinician, who may feel frustrated because of a desire to treat actively to a successful termination of therapy in a year; in such cases, the clinic administrator may face the difficult task of resolving, on an individual basis, the problem of the patients' overutilization of services.

Also part of the network are two community support centers, operated by staff from state, county, and voluntary agencies. They provide long-term day programs, social rehabilitation, psychotherapy, crisis intervention, and medication to the more severely impaired patients—those whose baseline of functioning is lower, who have been hospitalized more frequently, and who are less able to benefit from a more intensive, crisis-focused program. Dovetailing with the community support centers' programs is the Jawonio sheltered workshop, operated by the Rockland County Center for the Physically Handicapped; it provides prevocational and vocational training for psychiatrically disabled, physically handicapped, and some mentally retarded clients. Forty-seven of our group are currently served by the centers or the workshop.

In 1979 the Rockland center began the Growth Advancement Program as a specific response to the needs of young adult chronic patients. Operating as

We have had mixed success in ensuring that our young chronic patients actually use the services available to them. The crisis service is a typical point of entry to the system.

part of the community support centers, it offers such patients an opportunity to socialize and share problems with others their age. The program is designed to help young patients acquire the skills necessary to develop a system of community support and contacts outside the agency.

This is only the beginning of our response to the young adult chronic patient, and we are acutely aware of the need for new initiatives. We should note, however, that 25 per cent of our group (75 patients) have never been hospitalized; another 14 per cent (40 patients) have been hospitalized only once; 16 per cent (47 patients) have been hospitalized twice; and 45 per cent (132 patients) have been hospitalized three or more times.

While this low rate of hospitalization is gratifying insofar as it may reflect the effectiveness of our outpatient programs, it also has another consequence: a problem in meeting the need for case management services. We have in Rockland County, as part of the community support system, a program of case management services designed for patients who need help in handling activities of their daily lives and in maintaining their connection with treatment programs. For many of our young chronic patients, the relationship with the case manager is crucial to maintaining their functioning in times of stress—for example, when they lose a room or job and need a swift, helpful response from a trusted person.

Thirty-one per cent, or 90, of our group are receiving case management services. Sixty-three per cent of the 294, or 185 individuals, do not have a case manager. (For the remaining 6 per cent, the presence or absence of a case manager was undetermined.) While we do not know specifically why each of the 63 per cent lacks a case manager, we do know that 55 per cent are not eligible for case management because they are not eligible for the services of the community support system according to New York State criteria: three ten-day hospitalizations or three months' cumulative hospitalization within the past two years, or six months' consecutive hospitalization in a lifetime. Obviously, these criteria must be reconsidered if we are to provide more functionally disabled patients with case management and other vital services supported by community support system funds.

IS IT WORKING?

We asked our clinicians to indicate whether our present treatment and service programs were meeting the needs of young adult chronic patients. Their clinical judgment was that for 68 per cent of these patients, treatment needs are currently being met in the community, and that for 70 per cent, financial needs are being met. The clinicians' assessment is gratifying as far as it goes. But there remains a sizable minority whose treatment and financial needs are not being met, according to clinicians' assessments, or for whom the answer is unknown.

We also sought clinicians' judgments of the need for residential programs. They believed that 42 per cent of the group (122 patients) need a crisis residence occasionally. In spite of this considerable need, no crisis residence beds have been available to our patients because of state-imposed freezes on hiring staff for the community support system. Thirty-two per cent (95 patients) are seen as needing long-term residential treatment—again, too many for our county's one residential program of 20 beds.

NEED FOR RESIDENTIAL PROGRAMS

There is a crying need for residential programs for our young adult chronic population. In addition to those 217 perceived as needing a supportive place to live, either continually or on occasion, there may be a good number of others who would benefit from a residential program tailored to their needs, but who are instead living with their families as dependent children. The alternative, for those who cannot cope with single-room-occupancy hotels, is usually the proprietary home, in which middle-aged and elderly deinstitutionalized patients predominate, and where these younger patients are likely to feel that their despair of the future is confirmed.

The staff of our center, especially inpatient staff involved in discharge planning, see a need to test out residential programs with a supportive staff and well-defined structure, designed specifically to meet the developmental needs of young adults and to mesh with their treatment programs. Such residences could offer a refuge separated from the repetitive tragedies of family life and the accumulated weight of failed expectations. The hitherto impossible task of young adult development could be, if not completed, at least addressed with some consistency and hope for progress. Such residences could play a valuable role in ensuring continuity of care.

Such residences might also serve as locus and agent of real changes in family dynamics. They could offer, on the one hand, a realistic alternative to perpetual care of young patients by their parents. On the other hand, they might include family treatment to help parents to deal with their own sense of frustration and failure and to relate to their offspring in a way that encourages rather than impedes the process of separation. We

The creation of residential programs on a sufficient scale means overcoming some formidable obstacles: community resistance to neighborhood residences, and the more fundamental problem of funding.

cannot really expect families to "let go" until their impaired sons and daughters have somewhere else to go besides the street.

The creation of residential programs on a scale sufficient to make some impact means addressing and overcoming some formidable obstacles. One, of course, is community resistance to dealing with our young chronic patients in neighborhood residences, rather than as troublesome but isolated individuals wandering the streets. Another more fundamental problem is funding, both for residences and for other community mental health programs.

FUNDING NEW PROGRAMS

There is still a severe discrepancy in most states between the location of patients and the allocation of public mental health funds. In most cases the money to provide patient care has not followed patients from the state hospitals to the community systems that are now responsible for their treatment. While the massive discharge of patients, diversion of admissions, and policy of brief hospitalization have resulted in a dramatic reduction of census for most state hospitals, many hospitals now have larger budgets, even corrected for inflation, than they did ten or 20 years ago. Publicly funded community mental health systems, on the other hand, have not been granted the increase in funding required to provide clinical and social support to the older deinstitutionalized population, let alone our large and growing group of young adult chronic patients.

This discrepancy must be corrected, and it is up to us as administrators and clinicians to advocate reallocations of funds, pressing for changes in state legislatures and departments of mental health so that more effective treatment and residential programs in the community can be supported by adequate funding. While it has been fashionable until recent years for mental health professionals to eschew activist roles in the political process, we cannot continue to wait for others to demand the resources needed to ensure good patient care.

State and federal courts, in numerous right-to-treatment cases, have proven they can accomplish a great deal in reducing hospital populations and retaining patients in our communities, but they have been unsuccessful so far in guaranteeing monetary support for necessary community programs. While test cases that address the need for improvement of community resources might be encouraged, we cannot passively await these developments. Nor can we expect patients to press successfully for the additional money needed for their care. Demanding funds is up to us, and is fundamental to the development of new programs.

The work of developing more effective ways to meet the needs of our young adult chronic patients will be a major challenge in the coming decade. It is a challenge that, in social and human terms, we cannot afford to refuse.■

REFERENCES

1) National Institute of Mental Health, in *World Almanac and Book of Facts, 1981*, Newspaper Enterprise Association, New York City, 1980.

2) E. M. Gruenberg, "On the Pathogenesis of the Social Breakdown Syndrome," in *A Critical Review of Treatment Progress in a State Hospital Reorganized Toward the Communities Served: Treatment Programs, Present and Planned, of the Colorado State Hospital*, Colorado State Hospital, Pueblo, Colorado, 1963, pp. 96–108 (mimeograph).

3) E. M. Gruenberg, S. Brandon, and R. V. Kasius, "Identifying Cases of the Social Breakdown Syndrome," *Milbank Memorial Fund Quarterly*, Vol. 44, January 1966 (part 2), pp. 150–155.

4) S. Brandon and E. M. Gruenberg, "Measurement of the Incidence of Chronic Severe Social Breakdown Syndrome: Has the Dutchess County Service Been Associated With a Decline in Incidence?" *Milbank Memorial Fund Quarterly*, Vol. 44, January 1966 (part 2), pp. 129–149.

5) E. M. Gruenberg, "Can the Reorganization of Psychiatric Services Prevent Some Cases of Social Breakdown?" in *Psychiatry in Transition, 1966–67*, A. B. Stokes, editor, University of Toronto Press, Toronto, 1968, pp. 95–109.

6) E. M. Gruenberg, "The Social Breakdown Syndrome: Some Origins," *American Journal of Psychiatry*, Vol. 123, June 1967, pp. 1481–1489.

7) E. M. Gruenberg, H. B. Snow, and C. L. Bennett, "Preventing the Social Breakdown Syndrome," in *Social Psychiatry: Proceedings of the Association for Research in Nervous and Mental Disease, December 1–2, 1967, New York, New York*, F. C. Redlich, editor, Williams & Wilkins, Baltimore, 1969, pp. 179–195.

8) E. M. Gruenberg, D. M. Turns, S. P. Segal, *et al.*, "Social Breakdown Syndrome: Environmental and Host Factors Associated With Chronicity," *American Journal of Public Health*, Vol. 62, January 1972, pp. 91–94.

9) E. M. Gruenberg, "The Social Breakdown Syndrome and Its Prevention," in *American Handbook of Psychiatry: Volume II. Child and Adolescent Psychiatry, Sociocultural and Community Psychiatry*, 2nd edition, G. Caplan, editor, Basic Books, New York City, 1974, pp. 697–710.

10) E. Goffman, *Asylums: Essays on the Social Situation of Mental Patients and Other Inmates*, Aldine, Chicago, 1962.

11) C. L. M. Caton, "The New Chronic Patient and the System of Community Care," *Hospital & Community Psychiatry*, Vol. 32, July 1981, pp. 475–478.

12) G. G. Neffinger, "The Evolution of an Acute Day Treatment Program," *Hospital & Community Psychiatry*, Vol. 31, December 1980, pp. 826–828.

The New Chronic Patient: Clinical Characteristics of an Emerging Subgroup

STUART R. SCHWARTZ, M.D.
Director of Postgraduate Education
Department of Psychiatry
STEPHEN M. GOLDFINGER, M.D.
Medical Director
Psychiatric Emergency Services
San Francisco (Calif.) General Hospital

A subgroup of chronic mentally ill persons who have had little or no state hospitalization and who are difficult to engage in existing systems of community care is emerging in major urban areas. Observations made at a large municipal general hospital indicate the patients are typically young, more likely to be male, and highly transient. They have frequent interactions with emergency psychiatric and crisis units, coupled with intermittent involuntary short-term stays in local inpatient units. They have few skills and virtually no natural support systems. Under stress they show disorders in reality testing, exhibit anger and depression, and are prone to impulsive aggressive and self-destructive behaviors. They are typically unwilling to voluntarily accept continuing care. There is a lack of fit between this group's characteristic style of interaction and existing community-based programs. The costs of this lack of fit, both in staff morale and inappropriate use of expensive services, make the exploration of approaches to these "new chronic patients" a matter of immediate importance.

■Much of the literature on chronic care has emphasized a particular type of patient: a former state hospital resident now discharged into the community. Given years of deinstitutionalization in such states as California, New York, and Massachusetts, however, local mental health systems have been seeing persons who have seldom if ever been hospitalized in state facilities, but who have repeatedly been seen in acute services within the community. A few recent reports have addressed the difficulties with this emerging subgroup of the chronic mentally disabled (1–3).

Dr. Schwartz is also an associate clinical professor and Dr. Goldfinger is an assistant clinical professor at the School of Medicine of the University of California, San Francisco. Dr. Schwartz' address is Department of Psychiatry, San Francisco General Hospital, 1001 Potrero Avenue, San Francisco, California 94110. This paper is part of a series of four papers on the new chronic patient, which begins on page 463.

In this paper, we will first consider the clinical characteristics, diagnostic and behavioral features, and ego deficits of this subgroup. Next we will explore the problems that these patients pose when they interact with local mental health systems, especially in emergency and crisis intervention services. The impressions we present are a result of clinical observations over the past two years in San Francisco General Hospital, a large municipal hospital. We will begin by presenting a case report on an individual who represents a prototype of the new chronic patient.

CASE ILLUSTRATION

Mr. R is a 27-year-old white male who was brought into the psychiatric emergency services by the police after he was found wandering in traffic. Police said he appeared intoxicated and angry, yelling at them to mind their own business. His angry behavior persisted at the emergency services.

Mr. R is well known to the psychiatric emergency services. He has been seen eight times and hospitalized three times during the last year. The bulk of these appearances followed minor self-destructive acts (superficial wrist lacerations and minor drug overdoses) after which he was picked up by the police and admitted on an involuntary hold. During several visits he was intoxicated on alcohol, marijuana, or both; on one occasion he was flagrantly delusional following ingestion of PCP (phencyclidine).

After three of the more serious suicide gestures, he was hospitalized on the inpatient unit. Once he was referred to a halfway house but was discharged four days later for drinking. On another occasion he was referred to a day care program but dropped out after three days "Because I don't belong with those crazies."

On a third occasion a discouraged inpatient staff member referred him to the local outpatient clinic. After two visits he began missing scheduled appointments and dropping in at odd times. When his therapist was unable to see him during one of these drop-in visits, he screamed at the secretary that no one really cared, knocked over a vase, and walked out. Mr. R is a bitter and angry man who feels that the mental health system can't help him.

The patient grew up in a small town in central Florida. As a child he was a frequent runaway, and at age 12 his parents requested a foster home placement by the courts. At age 16 he ran away from the third of those placements to Miami, where he worked for some time as a dishwasher. At age 18 he met a young woman at a bar, and they took an apartment together. He described this time as "the happiest in my life; she cared." During this period, he worked at a parking lot while she worked as a waitress. He recalls drinking occasionally and smoking marijuana with some regularity but denies use of any other drugs then.

After a year the young woman became pregnant; when she told him, he felt that she had probably been cheating on him, became enraged, broke up their apartment, and left. On that occasion he made his first suicidal gesture by lacerating his wrist and was hospitalized briefly on a local inpatient unit.

After his discharge he moved to New Orleans, feeling that he had to get away from Florida and "all it stood for." In New Orleans he became more significantly involved in the drug subculture: he used amphetamines, barbiturates, and psychedelics and on a few occasions subcutaneously injected heroin. Although he worked at odd jobs, most of his income was provided by panhandling and petty shoplifting. He was arrested twice for petty theft and served brief jail sentences. During this period he began to feel that he was "hopeless" and made two additional suicide gestures.

At age 24 Mr. R moved to San Francisco. Since then he has supported himself on Social Security disability payments, and has lived in single-room-occupancy hotels in San Francisco's Tenderloin district. He described several intense but short-lived relationships. Although he has occasionally been able to work at minor jobs for a few months at a time, they have grown less frequent. His use of intoxicants increased and his depression deepened over the last year.

Mr. R is clearly a severely disturbed individual. His history and presentation evidence a long-standing pattern of impulsive and self-destructive behavior. With the possible exception of his years in Miami, his life seems devoid of any stable living situation or sustained interpersonal contact. His story seems to be one of overwhelming feelings of rage and depression. Even by running away or escaping into drugs or alcohol, he still cannot avoid these feelings.

Unable to ask for help directly, he engages in self-destructive behavior which, when discovered, ensures him access to immediate emergency intervention. However, his basic lack of trust precludes his following through on any voluntary treatment options. Angry and disappointed, he denies his own contributions to the problem, accusing and chastising the very clinicians whose help he has (albeit indirectly) secured. In response, the clinicians tend to become confused and angry by his repeated demands for and then rejections of their assistance, and frustrated by their inability to engage him in any meaningful therapeutic interaction.

EPIDEMIOLOGICAL CHARACTERISTICS

The group of patients represented by the case above are generally young, predominantly male, single, and unemployed. They appear to show a pattern of short-term, isolated residences with frequent moves within and between major cities. An analysis of patients seen in the psychiatric emergency services of San Francisco General Hospital from October to December 1980 produced the following data.[1] A review of every third patient seen (426 patients) revealed that 10.1 per cent of the patients were given a primary diagnosis of personality disorder, of which 67 per cent were seen as borderline (the most characteristic diagnosis for this group). A chart review of every patient so diagnosed and treated during October 1980 (N = 41) showed that 80 per cent of these patients were male, 90 per cent were under 35 years old, and 90 per cent were unemployed. Sixty-eight per cent were never married, with an additional 22 per cent either divorced or separated.

These new chronic patients are frequently transient members of large urban communities. In a study of 420 randomly selected patients seen in the same emergency services and similarly diagnosed, 20.9 per cent were found to have no regular local residence.[2] An additional 53.5 per cent claimed residence in a district of San Francisco noted to have no single-family residential homes, with 89 per cent of the residences hotel rooms or "studio apartments." Two-thirds of the residents of this area live alone or "with unrelated persons" (4).

Segal and co-workers have developed the concept of "social margin," defined as "all personal possessions, attributes, or relationships which can be traded on for help in time of need" (5). Individuals in this subgroup, who may be aggressive, manipulative, or withdrawing, have lost this currency, have run out of social margin. They have no remaining natural support systems, as they have alienated or isolated themselves from family, friends, or other social groups used in times of crisis. Consequently, community mental health services are often forced to assume this role during the recurring crisis in these patients' lives.

EGO DEFICITS

This population evidences a wide range of ego deficits. In particular, there are characteristic defects in reality testing, impulse control, and affective modulation. However, the extent to which these defects dominate the clinical picture, and the degree to which they incapacitate the patient, appears widely variable. More-

[1]Data in this section are from L. Chafetz, *Homelessness and Psychiatric Symptoms*, unpublished study, Department of Community and Mental Health Nursing, University of California, San Francisco, and S. Goldfinger and B. Havassy, Division of Program Evaluation, Department of Psychiatry, San Francisco General Hospital.

[2]L. Chafetz, *Homelessness and Psychiatric Symptoms*, unpublished study, Department of Community and Mental Health Nursing, University of California, San Francisco.

over, the behavior and level of functioning of a given patient appear to fluctuate dramatically over time, with profound implications for diagnosis and treatment decisions as well as for involuntary commitment procedures.

Deficiencies in the patients' reality testing are intermittent and occur under stress. Their thinking frequently has a paranoid character, but frank delusions and hallucinations are uncommon. They do not show the cognitive deficits associated with classic chronic schizophrenic disorders. Perceptions that contradict acceptable self- or object-images may be distorted or denied transiently. This distortion or denial may lead to an impression of discontinuity and chaotic disorganization in the patient's history.

The patients experience events as discontinuous. They seem to respond *de novo*, with no apparent ability to integrate a particular occurrence into a cohesive pattern. Judgment is often severely impaired. Plans and decisions may take on an overly unsubstantiated personalized meaning. Minor mishaps and losses may become distorted and magnified, crippling their ability to perceive and plan adaptive action.

Disorders of impulse control are prominent and are probably the most frequent precipitant of psychiatric intervention. Suicidal gestures and threats and other physically self-damaging acts are common. Although such patients less frequently direct major impulsive acts against other persons, they may have a history of involvement with the criminal justice system for low-level offenses such as minor property damage and petty assault. Episodic alcoholic intoxications as well as polydrug-abuse are frequent findings. Use of intoxicants tends to increase during periods of crisis.

Disturbances of affect are among the most notable features of this group. Anger and rage often predominate in the clinical picture, and the patients are frequently hostile, sarcastic, and argumentative. Within the treatment setting, this anger is often dramatically displayed, with shouting and minor property damage. It may appear to engulf everyone or everything in the patients' world, or be expressed only as sarcasm and disdain. In some patients, however, anger appears to be self-directed, replaced by helplessness and depression, which typically has an anhedonic quality. A sense of emptiness, alienation, and detachment from sources of pleasure and stimulation is a common complaint of these patients.

ASSESSMENT AND DIAGNOSIS

The clinical features and behavior patterns of this group frequently lead to marked difficulty in accurate diagnosis and assessment. All too frequently, charts document multiple contacts over an extended period of time, with different diagnostic classifications at each contact. Thus, for example, Chafetz found that 40 per cent of those patients diagnosed as borderline personalities who were seen for a second time during a three-month period were given a different diagnosis at the second visit.[3]

Because this group tends to use mental health services largely during periods of intense crisis, the evaluation of their level of functioning often reflects only their least integrated states. At times, indeed, they appear to function at a psychotic level, and provisional diagnoses such as brief reactive psychosis and schizophreniform or schizophrenic psychosis are made. In other situations, the affective picture may dominate, so that depressive diagnoses are also common.

The concomitant presence of drug or alcohol intoxication at presentation often further distorts the symptom picture. Many of this group are involved in the regular or intermittent use of psychoactive drugs (sometimes obtained illicitly) but maintain sufficient control of their use to avoid long-term addiction. Nevertheless, they can be mislabeled as drug-dependent, when in fact their use of drugs is really masking underlying deficits.

For patients who appear at the same facility on multiple occasions, thereby giving the interviewer greater opportunity to formulate a longitudinal view, a picture of severe character pathology begins to emerge. In many cases, these patients seem to exhibit some of the characteristics described under a variety of the personality disorders along axis 2 of *DSM-III*, but do not fall comfortably within any one personality disorder. A broader concept of *severe* borderline pathology would best characterize this group.

UTILIZATION OF SERVICES

Robbins describes a group of "unwelcome patients" who "cannot adapt to the community but cannot remain in the hospital" (3). Often they are left homeless when their hotel or boarding home casts them out for unacceptable behavior. Impulsive, aggressive, and self-destructive threats and behavior frequently bring these individuals to the attention of the police. Their entry into the system is often on an involuntary basis. The resultant intervention may take place within the mental health or the criminal justice system.

The specific characteristics of this patient group effectively preclude their appropriate utilization of many currently existing mental health services, including emergency psychiatric and crisis intervention services, inpatient hospitalization, residential treatment, and outpatient services.

Unfortunately, many aspects of the classic model of emergency intervention are grossly inappropriate for this population. For example, family support is often cited as an aid in the treatment of acute crisis situations. But these patients, largely estranged from their families, are often unwilling or unable to turn to family during periods of crisis. Indeed, the notion of invoking the help of environmental support systems for this population—where, as we have noted, the "social margin" is so narrow—is frequently useless.

Furthermore, emergency psychiatric care hinges on the assessment of the patient's level of functioning and chief complaint in order to establish the diagnosis and formulate an appropriate treatment plan and disposition. The very nature of the pathology of many of these patients precludes such an approach. Assessments relying on the patient's chief complaint on admission are hardly appropriate. In fact, the crisis at presentation is rarely the problem at all. The true source of difficulty is the enduring pattern of maladaptive living rather than the individual event that may precipitate a specific visit to a treatment facility.

Often the patients' self-description may appear grossly inconsistent. The history they give is unreliable. Pseudonyms are often used to mask previous visits. Their intra- and intercity mobility and transiency frequently preclude effective tracking. Thus specifics of past history, prior therapeutic involvements, and other relevant data are not available to the very emergency services that act as their primary care facility.

Within the emergency services, these patients, frequently brought in involuntarily, are often angry, demanding, hostile, and uncooperative (6). Their behavior toward the interviewer and their affective state may shift dramatically during an interview, often leading the interviewer to conclude that their requests are manipulative or illogical. Although they begin by dependently begging for whatever interventions the clinician can offer, they may disdainfully reject any treatment plan proposed. Such behavior may further alienate or confuse the emergency therapist, leading to feelings of impotence and anger and the wish to reject the patient.

Although talking to the clinician may serve a cathartic function or help the patients organize and recompensate sufficiently to return to their external environment, such interaction rarely has significant impact on ongoing functioning. Such patients frequently blame an external world, which they view as hostile and rejecting, for their problems. They are unable to incorporate any insight about the role that they play in creating and sustaining the stresses and crises of their lives. Although psychopharmacological interventions may aid in the management of such patients during periods of uncontrolled anxiety and rage, they have little effect on their basic maladaptive pattern.

On many occasions, self-destructive or impulsive behavior, quasi-delusional ideation, or the presence of drugs or alcohol intoxication that impede a diagnostic evaluation make it necessary for the emergency room clinician to look for a more protective ongoing treatment site, such as an inpatient unit. But inpatient hospitalization, so frequently employed as a means of stabilization and integration for the schizophrenic patient in exacerbation, has its own set of difficulties with the new chronic population (7).

Despite such patients' expressed wish to be protected and cared for during the initial phase of admission, they may feel threatened or overwhelmed by the stimulation level and intense interpersonal interaction of an inpatient environment. When attempts are made to use legal means to hold the patient for treatment beyond the acute emergency, they exercise a paradoxical capacity to regain control, and pull themselves together enough to avoid continued involuntary hospitalization.

Frequently unresponsive to psychotropic medication and unwilling to participate in individual and group psychotherapy, they may become hostile and belligerent on the ward. Inpatient staff become frustrated and are frequently anxious to discharge such patients as soon as they demonstrate a minimal functional capability. Thus they are sent out only to return to the emergency room of the same or another facility in a short time.

Outpatient referral is predicated on a patient's continued motivation to seek help for problems. Since many of these patients are unable to recognize the part they play in causing their ongoing difficulties, they frequently refuse to participate in such a referral. Those who do make a linkage with a traditional outpatient department fail to keep scheduled appointments, drop in at unusual times, and seem unable to follow through even when the therapist is patient, experienced, and concerned.

Finally, placement in residential facilities is often precluded by the very behaviors we might wish to treat. Given the patients' frequent history of drug abuse, alcoholism, self-destructive behavior, and acting out, typical halfway houses and other residential placements are unwilling to accept many of these patients.

STAFF ATTITUDES AND RESPONSES

One of the highest "costs" of the current pattern of interaction with these patients is the response of the caretakers themselves. As patients alternately demand and reject care, as they alternate between dependency, manipulation, withdrawal, anger, depression, and other interactive styles and emotional states, even the most tolerant and resourceful clinician is likely to experience increasing anger, bitterness, frustration, and helplessness. These responses, in turn, can lead to even more inappropriate treatment decisions, which are not in anyone's long-term interests but only serve to remove the patient, temporarily, from the responsibility of a given caretaker.

Adequate inservice education and training can help caretakers better understand the particular characteristics and psychodynamics of this subgroup, as well as their own responses to encounters with them. When the stresses of working with these patients are acknowledged, programs can take some steps to ensure either that specially trained and motivated workers are assigned to them, or that responsibility for their care is equitably dispersed among individual staff members. Ultimately, however, until staff have the programmatic tools to make some headway with this emerging population, it is unlikely that their effective burden will diminish.

FUTURE PROGRAM DEVELOPMENT

The above description and analysis is based on preliminary data from patients seen in one large municipal general hospital. It is clear that further empirical research and analysis are needed to provide a more precise and comprehensive picture of the characteristics of this emerging subgroup, of their interactions with a variety of community mental health services, and of the consequences of these interactions.

Nevertheless, our own experiences and those reported by colleagues in other communities clearly point out the lesson: there is an emerging, and apparently growing, subgroup of patients who are, in fact, chronically mentally ill, but who depart in significant ways from the traditional image of the chronic, formerly hospitalized patient.

All too often, they are handled by expensive acute care units, treated briefly with poor results. Even when the long-term nature of their pathology is acknowledged, existing service delivery systems seem unable to engage them appropriately. The patients do not see themselves as in need of help between their intermittent acute episodes, and therefore do not seem to fit into services, such as community support programs, built upon a comprehensive, voluntary rehabilitative model of care. As Bachrach has noted, "The planning of services for the chronically mentally ill represents a search for equilibrium among four competing sets of needs: those of the patient, the practitioner, the program, and the community" (8).

It is clear that addressing the needs of this emerging subgroup of chronic patients in a clinically appropriate and cost-effective manner poses a real challenge to mental health services, particularly in major urban areas. The group that we have described uses multiple modalities of services in both public and private sectors in an intermittent, unpredictable fashion. Therefore, the records available to clinicians reflect only part of the clinical picture.

Thus, a critical component of service delivery is a capacity to provide workers at these sites with sufficient background information on presenting individuals to permit appropriate diagnostic and treatment planning decisions. That implies the development of an ethical and effective patient tracking system. The technology for such an information system exists, but resistance to using that technology rests on real ethical issues rather than just on fiscal concerns. Nevertheless, we must attempt to devise a responsive and responsible information system that respects the rights and needs of patients (8).

In order to prevent the continued inappropriate and expensive use of services at the acute end of the spectrum, we must develop new models of service, with well-defined and realistic objectives, to fit the characteristic behavior patterns of this subgroup of chronic patients. Without careful data collection, we cannot document what happens to many of the patients between acute episodes. Longitudinal outcome studies that demonstrate the efficacy of existing interventions must be carried out as a preliminary step to any future planning.

Finally, we must explore the role of long-term hospitalization in the care of these patients. In changing the locus of care from state hospitals to communities, we have substantially reduced our willingness to provide long-term inpatient care to individuals for whom it may be the most appropriate and cost-effective service option. In their study of long- versus short-stay hospitalization, Glick and Hargreaves note that one result of long-term hospitalization was that such patients were more firmly engaged in the system of care after discharge (9).

This specific benefit would seem highly salient both to this patient group and to the local programs with which they interact. For it is not the needs of this emerging subgroup that distinguish them from other chronic patients. Rather, it is the problems attendant on their style of interaction with existing community-based services. At present, these "new chronic patients" are discontented, disengaged, and difficult for all who come in contact with them.■

REFERENCES

1) E. Bassuk and S. Gerson, "Chronic Crisis Patients: A Discrete Clinical Group," *American Journal of Psychiatry*, Vol. 137, December 1980, pp. 1513–1517.

2) J. R. Neill, "The Difficult Patient," *Journal of Clinical Psychiatry*, Vol. 40, May 1979, pp. 209–212.

3) E. Robbins, M. Stern, L. Robbins, *et al.*, "Unwelcome Patients: Where Can They Find Asylum?" *Hospital & Community Psychiatry*, Vol. 24, January 1978, pp. 44–46.

4) *Final Report of the Tenderloin Ethnographic Research Project: A Project of Central City Hospitality House*, San Francisco, September 1978.

5) S. P. Segal, J. Baumohl, and E. Johnson, "Falling Through the Cracks: Mental Disorder and Social Margin in a Young Vagrant Population," *Social Problems*, Vol. 24, February 1977, pp. 387–400.

6) J. C. Perry and G. L. Klerman, "Clinical Features of Borderline Personality Disorder," *American Journal of Psychiatry*, Vol. 137, February 1980, pp. 165–173.

7) G. Adler, "Hospital Treatment of Borderline Patients," *American Journal of Psychiatry*, Vol. 130, January 1973, pp. 32–36.

8) L. L. Bachrach, "Planning Mental Health Services for Chronic Patients," *Hospital & Community Psychiatry*, Vol. 30, June 1979, pp. 387–393.

9) I. M. Glick and W. A. Hargreaves, *Psychiatric Hospital Treatment for the 1980s: A Controlled Study of Short Versus Long Hospitalization*, Lexington Books, Lexington, Massachusetts, 1979.

The New Chronic Patient and the System of Community Care

CAROL L. M. CATON, PH.D.
Director
Division of Community Services Evaluation
New York State Psychiatric Institute
New York, New York

Deinstitutionalization has created a new type of patient—the new young chronic—who has received most or all of his treatment during brief hospital stays and through extended contact with outpatient community care programs. A one-year study of 119 new chronic patients entering treatment in New York City between 1977 and 1979 casts light on their living arrangements, use of mental health services, social functioning, criminal activity, suicide attempts, and symptomatology.

■The obvious presence of the chronic mental patient on the streets and back alleys of our major cities frequently is cited as evidence that our current mental health policies aren't working as well as they should. Indeed, the allegation that the chronic mental patient has been inadequately served by our large public mental health systems has been widely discussed in both professional and lay circles.

Despite the fact that several small-scale experimental projects or "model programs" for chronic mental patients in community settings have been developed (1–4), there has been little study and evaluation of ongoing service delivery systems to guide policy and program development. Thus, although the system has been accused of being unresponsive to the needs of the chronic patient, gaps in services to specific groups of patients have not been systematically identified.

One such patient group is the so-called new chronic patient—those who from the onset of their illness have been treated during the era of deinstitutionalization. Their treatment experiences have consisted of brief inpatient care (days or weeks) followed by outpatient aftercare, in contrast to the long-term institutional treatment of the previous era. The experiences of the long-stay patients, many of whom are elderly, during and after their transfer from publicly operated mental institutions to nursing homes, board-and-care facilities, and other community living arrangements have been studied extensively (5–10). In contrast, little information has been gathered on the clinical and social characteristics and service use patterns of the new chronics.

The new chronic mental patient and the system of community care is the subject of this report, which is based on a one-year socioepidemiological study of chronic schizophrenics in New York City. This study was begun in 1977, before the development of the State Office of Mental Health's community-based program for chronic patients (11), modeled after the federally sponsored community support program. The chief goals of the study were to investigate the outcome of schizophrenic patients receiving community care and to devise guidelines for community support program development. This report focuses on a description of patient outcome in terms of clinical and social functioning in the community, inpatient and outpatient service use, and life style.

CHOOSING THE SUBJECTS

One hundred and thirty-four chronic patients with a hospital diagnosis of schizophrenia and a history of at least two previous hospitalizations were selected for the study. Data on the postdischarge course were available for 119, or 89 per cent, of the 134; hence 119 patients make up the sample for this paper.

Half the study patients came from the inpatient wards of the state hospital serving northern Manhattan and half from inpatient facilities located within each of northern Manhattan's catchment areas. A deliberate attempt was made to select the high-risk chronic patient.

The remarkable success in following 89 per cent of an inner-city, lower-class cohort of patients is the result of

Dr. Caton is also an assistant professor in the department of psychiatry at the Columbia University College of Physicians and Surgeons in New York City. Her address at the institute is 722 West 168th Street, New York, New York 10032. The author is indebted to Charlotte Muller, Ph.D., for the cost data presented in this report and to Roger L. Spitzer, M.D., for his help on the use of the Schedule for Affective Disorders and Schizophrenia for checking the validity of the hospital diagnoses. This paper is based on a presentation at a conference on "The Young Adult Chronic Patient: Clinical and Programmatic Issues" sponsored by the Rockland County Community Mental Health Center November 20–21, 1980, in Suffern, New York. It is part of a series of four papers on the new chronic mental patient, which begins on page 463.

the research procedure of obtaining data on each patient's personal network (family, friends, landlords, and therapists), and the continuity of contacts between patients and our interviewers in the community itself.

The group was young (the mean age was 34), and most patients first became ill after the policy of deinstitutionalization went into effect in the state in 1968. Patients were excluded from the study if they were also mentally retarded, or if they were blind, deaf, mute, or nonambulatory. The majority of patients had a history of multiple hospitalizations that were difficult to document because they took place in a variety of state, municipal, and voluntary inpatient facilities in the New York City region and elsewhere.

Most patients were from social classes 4 and 5 of Hollingshead's Index of Social Position (12). The sample primarily was American and West Indian black (63 per cent) and Hispanic (20 per cent). More than one-fifth of the study subjects migrated to New York City from the Caribbean area.

All patients were referred to outpatient programs in their catchment areas after discharge from the hospital. The system of community care in northern Manhattan is based in each hospital's psychiatric service, as is typical of many comprehensive mental health programs. Clinic-based aftercare treatment, tailored to individual needs, included medication maintenance, group and individual therapy, and day hospital care. No attempt was made to control or to manipulate the community treatment given to study subjects. Rather, a goal of the study was to examine naturally occurring patterns of care.

Patients were followed in the community by research interviewers trained for the study in the use of standardized rating scales to assess symptomatology and role functioning, specifically the Global Assessment Scale (13) and the Psychiatric Evaluation Form (14). Each interviewer acted like a caseworker in following a cohort of patients. Patient use of the hospital and community treatment programs and the adequacy of aspects of the physical and socioemotional environment were assessed with the Community Care Schedule, a new rating scale instrument developed for this study (15). Service use data was the basis for an analysis of costs of community care. Cost methodology, described elsewhere (16), is based on established rates of reimbursement set for each individual program.

To check the validity of the hospital diagnosis of schizophrenia, half the sample participated in an interview based on a modified Schedule for Affective Disorders and Schizophrenia (SADS) conducted by a research psychologist trained in the use of the approach (17). Of the 60 patients given a SADS interview, it was possible to diagnose 42. The major reason the remaining 18 could not receive a research diagnosis was their recent and past history of severe substance abuse, making a precise determination of onset of psychotic symptoms impossible in the absence of an organic causal agent. In most cases, such subjects could not provide adequate anamnestic data on events related to the onset of their symptoms.

Of the 42 with a research diagnosis, nine (21.4 per cent) were given a diagnosis other than schizophrenia. Two suffered from drug dependence, two from alcohol dependence, one from major depressive disorder, one from antisocial personality, two from other psychiatric disorders, and one from an unspecified functional psychosis. It is notable that of the "misdiagnosed" cases, a higher percentage were black (89 per cent versus 61 per cent for the sample as a whole) and single (56 per cent versus 73 per cent for the sample as a whole).

It is significant that all nine patients with a research diagnosis other than schizophrenia were treated with antipsychotic medications in the hospital and in the aftercare treatment phase. There were no major differences in clinical condition at discharge, number of rehospitalizations, or clinical and social functioning in the community during the follow-up year for this subgroup of patients compared with the sample as a whole.

THE STUDY'S FINDINGS

The outcome data gathered on the study subjects included suicides, criminal activity, symptoms of psychosis, use of mental health services, and social life in the community.

Suicides. There were five suicides during the study year, all of which occurred in the community. Patients who committed suicide were younger (they averaged 26 years) than the average for the study group as a whole. Four of the five first became ill in their teens and were unmarried at the time of death. All the suicides were living with family or were separating from their family when the death occurred.

The one-year suicide rate of 4.2 per cent is twice that reported by Stein and Test for a comparable time period (18). It is 210 times the one-year suicide rate of 55 per 250,000 population reported in two northern Manhattan police precincts, the area in which most study patients lived.[1]

Criminal activity. Thirty-five patients had contact with the criminal justice system during the study year, seven as victims of crime and 26 as perpetrators, according to their self-reports. The two remaining had contact on noncriminal matters. Fifteen patients were arrested 30 times for offenses ranging from disorderly conduct, drunkenness, and driving violations to assault, theft, and sexual assault. The sample's arrest rate of 25 per cent compares with a 3 per cent rate in the two local police precincts.[1] However, these findings should be interpreted with caution because we were not able to compare the crime found in this patient sample with that of the general population, controlling for factors such as age, race, sex, and social class.

Symptoms of psychosis. As previously noted, the Psychiatric Evaluation Form, a rating scale instrument based on a 20-minute semistructured interview similar to the traditional psychiatric interview, was used quarterly to

[1]Data supplied by New York City Police Department, July 1980.

assess mental status. The symptoms of hallucinations, grandiosity, inappropriate affect, suspicion-persecution, speech disorganization, and disorientation were classified as positive symptoms of schizophrenia. A score of three or greater on a scale of 1 (no symptoms) to 6 (severe symptoms) was deemed sufficient to declare the presence of psychosis.

According to this classification scheme, 61 per cent of the study patients had at least one psychotic symptom sometime during the study year, either at discharge or at one of the quarterly assessments. At any single assessment, however, the per cent found psychotic ranged from 33.6 to 46.4 per cent.

Use of mental health services. As noted, all study patients were referred for psychopharmacological treatment and various psychosocial therapies based in outpatient clinic settings. However, only 17 per cent complied fully with the prescribed treatment plan during the postdischarge year, according to their self-reports. Those who complied were significantly more likely to remain out of the hospital.

The one-year rehospitalization rate was 58 per cent, approximately that found in an untreated group in an earlier, unrelated study (19). Twenty-eight per cent of the patients had multiple hospitalizations during the study year. There were a total of 122 rehospitalizations. It should be noted that studies of brief hospitalization conducted since deinstitutionalization have reported rehospitalization rates of about 60 per cent over a two-year period (20–22).

The high rehospitalization rate is costly to the mental health delivery system and exists despite the ready availability of aftercare treatment services. For example, the mean cost of mental health services per case in our study was nearly four times higher for those patients hospitalized during the postdischarge year. The mean cost per case for the entire sample was $7,125; for those not hospitalized it was $2,690, but for those who were hospitalized it was $10,103. Ten per cent of the sample incurred mental health service costs that exceeded the cost of one year of continuous stay in a state facility, about $22,000.

Social life in the community. There is considerable evidence that the level of social functioning among the sample patients has declined since the onset of their illnesses. For example, although 89 per cent of study patients had once held a job, only 27 per cent worked during the study year. Twelve per cent worked full time for pay, but only one person worked full time for pay continuously throughout the year.

Virtually all the patients in the study group resided in natural living environments in the community. Forty-two per cent lived with their families, 24 per cent lived in single-room-occupancy hotels, and 28 per cent lived alone in their own apartments.

One quarter of the sample had been married at one time, and study patients had parented 48 children. Only about half the sample were rated as having social support, meaning the availability of someone other than a psychiatric professional to turn to in case of need. The majority of supporters lived in the same household as the patient (32 per cent), or in the same building or neighborhood (40 per cent).

It is significant that many patients were living with their families. Clinicians traditionally have relied heavily on family support in carrying out a community care policy. While family studies have shown that the presence of a mental patient in the family can be stressful (23,24), studies of brief hospitalization and community alternatives to hospitalization show evidence that early release or management of psychosis without hospitalization imposes little additional psychological burden on the family (18,25). However, those studies did not investigate the long-term impact of a policy of community placement on family structure.

In our study we found that 62.5 per cent of patients who had been married were divorced or separated at the time of discharge, that 72 per cent of patients who were parents were not living with their dependent children, and that 39 per cent of patients had severely limited contact with family. It is noteworthy that family care was rarely available to subjects in our study.

MOBILIZING FOR THE YOUNG CHRONIC

While it has long been known that social disability can be a sequela of the major functional psychoses, the extent of the new chronic patient phenomenon is an unanticipated consequence of the deinstitutionalization movement. Indeed, for years it was assumed that chronicity was caused largely by the custodial philosophy of public mental institutions, a thesis rendered some support by psychosocial studies of the mental hospital conducted in the 1950s (26–28). It was hoped that outpatient management of mental illness with minimal use of the psychiatric hospital would facilitate maintenance of social competence and involvement in the life of society at large. However, it is now widely recognized that the phasedown of the asylum will not eliminate chronicity. Intensified efforts must be made to better understand the determinants of chronicity regardless of the locus of care.

Our findings illustrate some critical issues in community treatment of the young adult new chronic patient. Even though the service systems under study provided what can be termed "state of the art" community programming, the excessively high rehospitalization rate, poor treatment compliance, and high level of symptomatology in the community indicate that the system is not working well for this patient group. There obviously is a need to develop innovative approaches to engage the patient in the long-term maintenance treatment that may be necessary for the rest of his life.

Although the extent of criminal behavior among ex-patients has been widely discussed and debated (29), our findings show that even when arrests are made, misdemeanors are far more common than felonies. The high suicide rate in the study reported here suggests that suicide may be a more significant problem in community management than crime. That finding, along with those of other studies of suicide among the seriously ill (30), suggests that the suicidal potential of patients released from the hospital must be carefully evaluated and continuously monitored.

Moreover, the young adult patient should be assisted to maintain his best level of social competence in key areas such as work, family and social relationships, and citizenship in the community. New ways of making use of the supportive potential of the natural living environment involving family, friends, landlords, neighbors, and traditional caregivers such as the clergy deserve exploration. Counseling for family members and significant others might enable them to cope more effectively with the chronic patient. Children of the young adult chronic patient, virtually ignored by our current delivery system, should be included in this process.

Finally, our future research efforts must teach us more about the causes of chronicity—biological, social, or both. A better understanding of the illness process is necessary for the mental health professions to mobilize the mental health delivery system to enable the young adult chronic patient to maintain maximum involvement in life.■

REFERENCES

1) M. A. Test and L. I. Stein, "Training in Community Living: Research Design and Results," in *Alternatives to Mental Hospital Treatment*, L. I. Stein and M. A. Test, editors, Plenum, New York City, 1978, pp. 57–74.

2) B. Pasamanick, F. Scarpitti, and S. Dinitz, *Schizophrenics in the Community: An Experimental Study of the Prevention of Hospitalization*, Appleton-Century Crofts, New York City, 1967.

3) L. R. Mosher, S. Matthews, and A. Menn, "Soteria: A New Treatment for Schizophrenia: One Year Follow-up Data," *American Journal of Orthopsychiatry*, Vol. 44, March 1974, pp. 207–208.

4) L. L. Bachrach, "Overview: Model Programs for Chronic Patients," *American Journal of Psychiatry*, Vol. 137, September 1980, pp. 1023–1031.

5) E. N. Gopelrud, "Unexpected Consequences of Deinstitutionalization of the Mentally Disabled Elderly," *American Journal of Community Psychology*, Vol. 7, June 1979, pp. 315–329.

6) K. F. Jasnau, "Individualized Versus Mass Transfer of Nonpsychotic Geriatric Patients From Mental Hospitals to Nursing Homes With Special Reference to the Death Rate," *Journal of the American Geriatrics Society*, Vol. 15, March 1967, pp. 280–284.

7) E. W. Markson and J. H. Cumming, "The Post-Transfer Fate of Relocated Mental Patients in New York," *Gerontologist*, Vol. 15, April 1975, pp. 104–108.

8) T. Pihkanen and M. Lahdenpera, "Observations on the Effects Produced by Hospital Transfer in a Group of Chronic Neuropsychiatric and Geriatric Patients," *Acta Psychiatrica Scandanavica*, Vol. 39, supplement 169, 1963, pp. 335–347.

9) E. Marks, M. Blenkner, M. Bloom, *et al.*, "Some Factors and Their Association With Post-Relocation Mortality Among Institutionalized Aged Persons," *Journal of Gerontology*, Vol. 27, No. 3, 1972, pp. 376–382.

10) J. P. Zweig and J. Z. Csank, "Mortality Fluctuations Among Chronically Ill Medical Geriatric Patients as an Indicator of Stress Before and After Relocation," *Journal of the American Geriatrics Society*, Vol. 24, June 1976, pp. 264–277.

11) J. Prevost and A. Arnold, *Five Year Plan for Community Placement and Support*, State of New York Office of Mental Health, Albany, January 1978.

12) A. B. Hollingshead, *The Two-Factor Index of Social Position*, privately published, New Haven, Connecticut, 1958.

13) J. Endicott, R. L. Spitzer, J. L. Fleiss, *et al.*, "The Global Assessment Scale: A Procedure for Measuring Overall Severity of Psychiatric Disturbance," *Archives of General Psychiatry*, Vol. 33, June 1976, pp. 766–771.

14) J. Endicott and R. L. Spitzer, "What! Another Rating Scale: The Psychiatric Evaluation Form," *Journal of Nervous and Mental Disease*, Vol. 154, February 1972, pp. 88–104.

15) C. L. M. Caton, C. Muller, and R. L. Spitzer, *The Community Care Schedule*, New York State Psychiatric Institute, New York City, 1981.

16) C. Muller and C. L. M. Caton, *Economic Cost of Schizophrenia: A Post-Discharge Study*, New York State Psychiatric Institute, New York City, 1981.

17) R. L. Spitzer and J. Endicott, "Schedule for Affective Disorders and Schizophrenia," in *Biometrics*, 3rd edition, New York State Psychiatric Institute, New York City, 1978.

18) M. A. Test and L. I. Stein, *An Alternative to Mental Hospital Treatment: II. Social Cost*, University of Wisconsin, Madison, 1978.

19) G. E. Hogarty, S. C. Goldberg, N. R. Schooler, *et al.*, "Drug and Sociotherapy in the Aftercare of Schizophrenic Patients," *Archives of General Psychiatry*, Vol. 31, November 1974, pp. 603–608.

20) M. I. Herz, J. Endicott, and R. L. Spitzer, "Brief Hospitalization of Patients With Families: Initial Results," *American Journal of Pychiatry*, Vol. 132, April 1975, pp. 413–418.

21) I. D. Glick, W. A. Hargreaves, M. Raskin, *et al.*, "Short Versus Long Hospitalization: A Prospective Controlled Study: I. Results for Schizophrenic Inpatients," *American Journal of Psychiatry*, Vol. 132, April 1975, pp. 385–390.

22) E. M. Caffey, C. R. Galbrecht, C. I. Klett, *et al.*, "Brief Hospitalization and Aftercare in the Treatment of Schizophrenia," *Archives of General Psychiatry*, Vol. 24, January 1971, pp. 81–86.

23) J. Grad and P. Sainsbury, "Mental Illness and the Family," *Lancet*, Vol. 1, March 9, 1963, pp. 544–547.

24) J. Grad and P. Sainsbury, "The Effects That Patients Have on Their Families in a Community Care and Control Psychiatric Service: A Two Year Follow-up," *British Journal of Psychiatry*, Vol. 114, January 1968, pp. 265–278.

25) M. I. Herz, J. Endicott, and R. L. Spitzer, "Brief Versus Standard Hospitalization: The Families," *American Journal of Psychiatry*, Vol. 133, July 1976, pp. 795–801.

26) E. Goffman, *Asylums: Essays on the Social Situation of Mental Patients and Other Inmates*, Anchor Books, Garden City, New York, 1964.

27) H. W. Dunham and H. K. Weinberg, *The Culture of the State Mental Hospital*, Wayne State University Press, Detroit, 1960.

28) A. H. Stanton and M. S. Schwartz, *The Mental Hospital*, Basic Books, New York City, 1954.

29) J. G. Rabkin, "Criminal Behavior of Discharged Mental Patients: A Critical Appraisal of the Research," *Psychological Bulletin*, Vol. 86, January 1979, pp. 1–27.

30) M. T. Tsuang, "Suicide in Schizophrenics, Manics, Depressives, and Surgical Controls," *Archives of General Psychiatry*, Vol. 35, February 1978, pp. 153–155.

COMMENTARY

YOUTHFUL CHRONICITY: PARADOX OF THE 80s

Young adult chronic patients challenge us. With a boldness characteristic of their youth, they reveal that serious, long-term mental illness exists, confounding our interventions. Continuously maladaptive in life style, they demonstrate that changing the locus of care from hospital to community does not, in and of itself, impact on chronicity.

The emergence of this problematic population is not, perhaps, a new configuration of illness, but the result of a combination of factors. Among them are the increased public visibility of the mentally ill, a byproduct of the deinstitutionalization movement, and their increased numbers, an end product of the post-World-War-II baby boom. Both their numbers and their resistance to our current treatment efforts force us to realize once again how much we still need to learn about the therapeutic, social, and economic aspects of chronic mental illness.

We do know that although these patients do not make up a diagnostically homogeneous population, they have certain characteristics in common. They have difficulty forming stable relationships and have little or no natural support systems. Socially and psychologically fragile, and often psychotic, they are acutely vulnerable to stress. They frustrate our treatment efforts, resist ongoing affiliation, and frequently choose a sporadic semi-involvement during recurring crisis periods in their lives.

Given this, can we continue to assume that the traditional responses to the problems of chronicity will be effective? These young adults provide ample evidence that they are not. How should we, therefore, understand the dynamics of chronicity, and which constructs and definitions have treatment value? What are the treatment modalities that will best serve the young adult chronic patient?

We also need to understand the impact these patients have upon the larger human service network. A recent survey of a shelter for homeless men in a large northeastern city contradicted the traditional profile of the elderly, uneducated, impoverished skid-row male resident. Rather, one-half were under age 35, and a fifth were in their 20s. Half had completed high school, and more than a fifth had attended college. Twenty per cent were found to have psychiatric disorders; in three-fourths they were of psychotic proportions. The fact that it is a city shelter that offers the mentally ill a haven from the street reveals the inadequacy of our current service system.

The homelessness of these young adults, and their involvement in a variety of low-level criminal activities and in substance abuse, frightens a society already burdened by its own increasing violence and raises questions of service provision. How can we reduce the fragmentation of the present human service delivery system? How do we provide support to the generic human service network, responding in ways that do not, as in the past, perpetuate the segregation of the mentally ill?

In this era of dwindling human service resources, mental health systems across the nation are confronted with a future in which growth over inflation appears unattainable. Therefore we must ask ourselves for which dysfunctions will this population require hospitalization, and for which will community-based treatment approaches be not only therapeutically sound, but cost-effective.

Seventy years ago, at a conference entitled, interestingly enough, "Arrest of Development in Adolescence," Adolf Meyer urged his colleagues to "turn from generalizing attitudes to conscientious observation and careful evaluation of actual facts." Is not this exhortation valid today as we seek solutions for a group of the mentally ill who are in peril?—James A. Prevost, M.D., *commissioner, New York State Office of Mental Health*